ECHINOCOCCOSIS

Edited by **Tonay Inceboz**

Echinococcosis
http://dx.doi.org/10.5772/65181
Edited by Tonay Inceboz

Contributors

Deniz Balci, Can Konca, Kiyoshi Kita, Shigehiro Enkai, Kimitoshi Sakamoto, Miho Kaneko, Hirokazu Kouguchi, Takao Irie, Kinpei Yagi, Jun Matsumoto, Yuzaburo Oku, Ken Katakura, Osamu Fujita, Tomoyoshi Nozaki, Yuka Ishida, YuRong Yang, Shukun Yang, Yumin Zhao, Donald McManus, Angeliki Vidoura, Tonay Inceboz

Published by InTech
Janeza Trdine 9, 51000 Rijeka, Croatia

Publishing Process Manager Edi Lipovic
Technical Editor SPi Global
Cover InTech Design team

First published November, 2017
Printed in Croatia
Legal deposit, Croatia: National and University Library in Zagreb

Additional hard copies can be obtained from orders@intechopen.com

Echinococcosis, Edited by Tonay Inceboz
p. cm.
Print ISBN 978-953-51-3591-3
Online ISBN 978-953-51-3592-0

For EU product safety concerns:
IN TECH d.o.o., Prolaz Marije Krucifikse Kozulić 3, 51000 Rijeka, Croatia,
info@intechopen.com or visit our website at intechopen.com.

Meet the editor

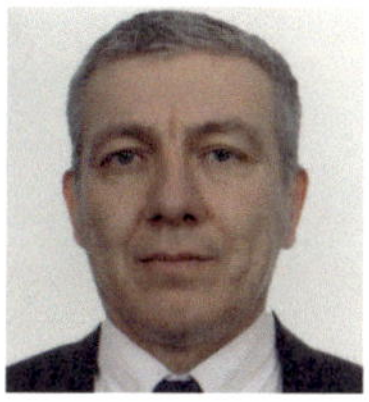

Tonay Inceboz, a senior lecturer in Medical Parasitology, has graduated from Ege University of Medical Faculty (Turkey) in 1988 and completed his Med. PhD degree in Medical Parasitology at the same university in 1998. He became an associate professor in 2008 and a professor in 2014. He is currently working as a professor in the Department of Medical Parasitology at Dokuz Eylul University, Izmir, Turkey. His main research interests are *Echinococcus granulosus, Echinococcus multilocularis* (diagnosis, life cycle, in vitro and in vivo cultivation), and *Trichomonas vaginalis* (diagnosis, PCR, and in vitro cultivation). He is married and has one daughter named Melody.

Contents

Preface

Echinococcosis is a major parasitic zoonotic infection caused by cestode of the *Echinococcus* species. There are four most common species: *E. granulosus*, *E. multilocularis*, *E. vogeli*, and *E. oligarthrus*. *Echinococcus* involves two hosts: a definitive host (carnivores such as dogs, wolves, and foxes) and an intermediate host (herbivores such as sheep, horses, cattle, pigs, goats, camels, moose, kangaroos, and humans). It is a public health importance worldwide.

The book has been organized into four major sections: (I) The Introduction section. (II) the diagnosis of echinococcosis is based on clinical findings, imaging, and serology. There are numerous diagnostic methods for lab diagnosis of echinococcosis, and in this book, you will find very motivating knowledge in *Current Research Advance on Echinococcosis* written by Shukun Yang et al.; (III) Therapy for echinococcosis depends on the size, location, and symptoms of the cysts and the overall health of the patient. There are medical and surgical approaches; however, medical approach—basically albendazole—is a neoadjuvant and adjuvant therapy. It reduces the risk of recurrent disease by the inactivation of the protoscolices. Surgery is the principle treatment modality. In this book, you will not only find the detailed information on surgical management including surgical complications contributed by Angeliki Vidoura et al. and Can Konca at al. (IV) but also new horizons for drug therapy written by Shigehiro Enkai et al. Section 2 includes topics covering *Echinococcus* species, interactions between parasites and hosts, and immunotherapy agents, including drug and vaccine discoveries. Section 3 includes topics covering the surgical management of echinococcosis, hydatid disease surgical approach, pericystectomy, cystic hepatic echinococcosis, hepatic hydatid cyst, open surgical approach, bile leakage, bile fistula, biliary complication, and prevention. Section 4 includes topics on the drug discovery, fumarate respiration, mitochondrial complex II, and ascofuranone.

In conclusion, worldwide well-known scientific people shared their valuable, updated knowledge on echinococcosis in this book. At this point, I want to express my sincere thanks to all authors for their great contributions and also to Mr. Edi Lipović for his kind support. I believe this book will lead to many scientific investigations in the future.

Tonay Inceboz, MD
Professor
Dokuz Eylul University, Medical Faculty,
Department of Parasitology, Turkey

Section 1

Introduction

Chapter 1

Introductory Chapter: Overview on Echinococcosis

Tonay Inceboz

Additional information is available at the end of the chapter

http://dx.doi.org/10.5772/intechopen.70583

1. Overview on echinococcosis

Echinococcosis is a zoonotic helminth disease. First, description goes back to 1684 when Francesco Redi has first described the scolex. Then, in 1700s, Philip Jacob Hartmann has defined in an adult form. Since intercontinental travelling is very common, it has been an important health problem in the last decades. Although it has been known for many years, it keeps its peculiarity [1–3].

Echinococcus belongs to Cestoda (class) and the Taeniidae (family). There are four most common species: *Echinococcus granulosus*, *Echinococcus multilocularis*, *Echinococcus vogeli* and *Echinococcus oligarthrus*. The most common one is *E. granulosus*, causing cystic echinococcosis (CE), whereas *E. vogeli* is the rarest species. *E. multilocularis* is also rare; however, it is the most violent species causing alveolar echinococcosis (AE). *E. vogeli* and *E. oligarthrus* cause polycystic echinococcosis (PE). There are other species of *Echinococcus*; *Echinococcus canadensis*, *Echinococcus equinus*, *Echinococcus ortleppi* and *Echinococcus shiquicus*. There are also many different genotypes of each species; *E. granulosus* has 10 genotypes (G1–G10), whereas *E. multilocularis* has two genotypes (M1–M2) [4, 5].

Echinococcosis is very widely distributed in all over the world; CE is found in North Pole, Asia, Europe, Africa, Australia and South America. AE is found in Alpine and sub-Arctic or Arctic regions, including Canada, the United States and Central and Northern Europe, China and Central Asia. PE is found in Central and South America [4, 6, 7].

Humans are not definitive hosts; however, two forms of echinococcosis important in humans are CE and AE. Although most people with the disease are asymptomatic, CE causes slowly growing cysts in the liver, lungs and other organs that can be undiagnosed for many years. AE, however, poses a much greater risk than CE, causing parasitic tumors in many organs and can be fatal, if left untreated [4, 6].

The diagnosis of echinococcosis is based on clinical findings, pathology, imaging and serology. There are numerous diagnostic methods for lab diagnosis of echinococcosis. The diagnosis of echinococcosis is based on clinical findings, imaging (radiology, ultrasonography, computed axial tomography, magnetic resonance imaging) [8, 9] and serology tests such as indirect hemagglutination (IHA) [10], enzyme-linked immunosorbent assay (ELISA), IgG-ELISA [11–13] or IgE-ELISA [14], immunoblotting (IB), Western blot 7 kDa and/or 18 kDa for CE and 28 kDa for AE [15] and *E. multilocularis* for diagnosis of Em2plus-ELISA [16], Em18 [17, 18], Em70 and Em90 [19]. On the other hand, various techniques such as random amplification of polymorphic DNA (PCR-RAPD), restriction fragment length polymorphism (PCR-RFLP) [20, 21] and multiplex PCR for a quick identification were used to determine genetic variations [22, 23].

Therapy for echinococcosis depends on the size, location and symptoms of the cysts and the overall health of the patient. There are medical and surgical approaches; however, medical approach—basically albendazole—is a neoadjuvant and adjuvant therapy. It reduces the risk of recurrent disease by the inactivation of the protoscolices. Surgery is the principle treatment modality [24, 25].

Author details

Tonay Inceboz

Address all correspondence to: tonay.inceboz@gmail.com

Medical Faculty, Department of Parasitology, Dokuz Eylul University, Turkey

References

[1] Redi F. Osservazioni intorno agli animal viventi che si trouvano negli animali viventi. Firenze: Piero Matini; 1684. p. 244

[2] David I. Grove. A History of Human Helminthology. Wallingford, Oxon: CAB International, 1990. p. viii + 848. ISBN: 0-85198-689-7. DOI:10.1017/S0007087400027965

[3] Craig PS, McManus DP, Lightowlers MW, Chabalgoity JA, Garcia HH, Gavidia CM, Schantz PM. Prevention and control of cystic echinococcosis. Lancet Infectious Diseases. 2007;**7**(6):385-394. DOI: 10.1016/S1473-3099(07)70134-2

[4] World Health Organization. About Echinococcosis. Available from: http://www.who.int/echinococcosis/about_disease/en/

[5] Alvarez Rojas CA, Romig T, Lightowlers MW. *Echinococcus granulosus* sensu lato genotypes infecting humans—Review of current knowledge. International Journal for Parasitology. 2014;**44**:9-18. DOI: 10.1016/j.ijpara.2013.08.008

[6] Sachar S, Goyal S, Sangwan S. Uncommon locations and presentations of hydatid cyst. Annals of Medical and Health Sciences Research. 2014;**204**:447-452. DOI: 10.4103/2141-9248.133476

[7] Hotez PJ, Gurwith M. Europe's neglected infections of poverty. International Journal of Infectious Diseases. 2011;**15**:e611-e619. DOI: 10.1016/j.ijid.2011.05.006

[8] Moro P. Clinical Manifestations and Diagnosis of Echinococcosis. UpToDate. Last updated 2017. Available from: http://www.uptodate.com/contents/clinical-manifestations-and-diagnosis-of-echinococcosis

[9] Inceboz T, Goktay Y, Sagol O, Korkmaz M, Uner A. Mesenteric Doppler ultrasonography findings of *Echinococcus multilocularis* infection: An experimental study. Türkiye Parazitolojii Dergisi. 2009;**33**(2):151-154 PubMed PMID: 19598092

[10] Auer H, St€ockl C, Suhendra S, Schneider R. Sensitivity and specificity of new commercial tests for the detection of specific Echinococcus antibodies. Wiener Klinische Wochenschrift. 2009;**121**:37e41. DOI: 10.1007/s00508-009-1233-4

[11] Zhang W, McManus DP. Recent advances in the immunology and diagnosis of echinococcosis. FEMS Immunology and Medical Microbiology. 2006;**47**:24e41. DOI: 10.1111/j. 1574- 695X.2006.00060.x

[12] Carmena D, Benito A, Eraso E. Antigens for the immunodiagnosis of *Echinococcus granulosus* infection: An update. Acta Tropica. 2006;**98**:74e86. DOI: 10.1016/j.actatropica.2006. 02.002

[13] Sarkari B, Rezaei Z. Immunodiagnosis of human hydatid disease: Where do we stand? World Journal of Methodology. 2015;**26**;**5**(4):185-195. DOI: 10.5662/wjm.v5.i4.185

[14] Lawn SD, Bligh J, Craig PS, Chiodini PL. Human cystic echinococcosis: Evaluation of post-treatment serologic follow-up by IgG subclass antibody detection. The American Journal of Tropical Medicine and Hygiene. 2004;**70**:329e335 PMID: 15031526

[15] Liance M, Janin V, Bresson-Hadni S, Vuitton AD, Houın R, Piarroux R. Immunodiagnosis of echinococcus infections: Confirmatory testing and species differentiation by a new commercial western blot. Journal of Clınical Microbiology. 2000;**38**(10):3718-3721 PMID: 11015390

[16] Gottstein B, Jacquıer P, Bresnon-Hadni S, Eckert J. Improved primary immunodiagnosis of alveolar echinococcosis in humans by an enzyme-linked Immunosorbent assay using the Em2Plus antigen. Journal of Clinical Microbiology. 1993;**31**(2):373-376 PMID: 8432825

[17] Bart JM, Piarroux M, Sako Y, Grenouillet Bresson-Hadni S, Piarroux R, Ito A. Comparison of several commercial serologic kits and Em18 serology for detection of human alveolar echinococcosis. Diagnostic Microbiology and Infectious Disease. 2007;**59**:93-95. DOI: 10.1016/j.diagmicrobio.2007.03.018

[18] Ito A, Xiao N, Liance M, Sato MO, Sako Y, Mamuti W, Ishikawa Y, Nakao M, Yamasaki H, Nakaya K, Bardonnet K, Bresson-Hadni S, Vuitton DA. Evaluation of an enzyme-linked immunosorbent assay (ELISA) with affinity-purified Em18 and an ELISA with recombinant Em18 for differential diagnosis of alveolar echinococcosis: Results of a blind test. Journal of Clinical Microbiology. 2002;**40**:4161e4165 PMID: 12409391

[19] Korkmaz M, Inceboz T, Celebi F, Babaoglu A, Uner A. Use of two sensitive and specific immunoblot markers, Em70 and Em90, for diagnosis of alveolar echinococcosis. Journal of Clinical Microbiology. 2004;**42**:3350e3352. DOI: 10.1128/JCM.42.7.3350-3352.2004

[20] Bowles J, McManus DP. Rapid discrimination of echinococcus species and strains using a polymerase chain reaction-based RFLP method. Molecular and Biochemical Parasitology. 1993;**57**:231e239 PMID: 8094539

[21] Xiao N, Nakao M, Qiu J, Budke CM, Giraudoux P, Craig PS, Ito A. Dual infection of animal hosts with different Echinococcus species in the eastern Qinghai-Tibet plateau region of China. The American Journal of Tropical Medicine and Hygiene. 2006;**75**:292e294 PMID: 16896135

[22] Boubaker G, Macchiaroli N, Prada L, Cucher MA, Rosenzvit MC, Ziadinov I, Deplazes P, Saarma U, Babba H, Gottstein B, Spiliotis M. A multiplex PCR for the simultaneous detection and genotyping of the *Echinococcus granulosus* complex. PLoS Neglected Tropical Diseases. 2013;**7**:e2017. DOI: 10.1371/journal.pntd.0002017

[23] Can H, Inceboz T, Caner A, Atalay Şahar E, Karakavuk M, Döşkaya M, Çelebi F, Değirmenci Döşkaya A, Gülçe İz S, Gürüz Y, Korkmaz M. Detection of *Echinococcus granulosus* and *Echinococcus multilocularis* in cyst samples using a novel single tube multiplex real-time polymerase chain reaction. Mikrobiyoloji Bülteni. 2016;**50**(2):266-277 Turkish PubMed PMID: 27175499

[24] McManus DP, Gray DJ, Zhang W, Yang Y. Diagnosis, treatment, and management of echinococcosis. British Medical Journal. 2012;**344**:e3866. PMID: 22689886. DOI: 10.1136/bmj.e3866

[25] Kern P. Clinical features and treatment of alveolar echinococcosis. Current Opinion in Infectious Diseases. 2010;**23**:505-512. DOI: 10.1097/QCO.0b013e32833d7516

Section 2

The Diagnosis of Echinococcosis

Chapter 2

Current Research Advance on Echinococcosis

Shukun Yang, Yumin Zhao,
Don Peter McManus and YuRong Yang

Additional information is available at the end of the chapter

http://dx.doi.org/10.5772/intechopen.68286

Abstract

Echinococcosis is caused by infection with larva (metacestode) of the tapeworms of the genus *Echinococcus*. Within genus *Echinococcus*, two species are known as public health concern worldwide: *Echinococcus guanulosus* causing cystic echinococcosis (CE) and *Echinococcus multilocularis* causing alveolar echinococcosis (AE). The co-evaluation due to the interaction between parasites and their hosts has been well known to be able to allow tolerating to maintain parasitism as long as possible. With many research advanced findings, scientists have been much interested in using either those molecules from parasites producing due to invading and surviving or those cytokines from hosts responding due to defenses to carry out immunotherapeutic practice that is not only against parasitic infection but also for cancer or other immunological related disorders. Taken advance of knowledge on *Echinococcus* genome research outcomes, recent attentions regarding the discoveries of targeting antiparasitic drug and/or vaccine were extensively discussed in this review.

Keywords: *Echinococcus* species, parasitism, interactions between parasites and hosts, immunotherapy agents, drug and vaccine discoveries

1. Introduction

The echinococcosis in human occurs as a result of infection by the larval stages of taeniid cestodes of the genus *Echinococcus*. Originally, four species have been recognized as the public health concern: *Echinococcus granulosus* [agent of cystic echinocococcosis (CE)], *Echinococcus multilocularis* [agent of alveolar echinococcosis (AE)], and *Echinococcus vogeli* and *Echinococcus oligarthrus* [both are the agents of polycystic echinococcosis (PE)] [1]. Recently, two new species have been identified: *Echinococcus shiquicus* [2] in small mammals from the Tibetan plateau and *Echinococcus felidis* [3] in African lions though these two new species infective to human are still unknown [4]. A couple of studies have provided augments that these diseases are an increasing public health concern and showing emerging or re-emerging diseases [4, 5].

Among recognized four public health concerned species, *E. multilocularis* and *E. granulosus* are important for human health and economic welfare [4]. The disease occurs in most areas of the world, and currently about 4 million people are infected and another 40 million people are at risk [4, 6, 7]. The economic cost of the disease is estimated to be around 3 billion USD a year. It is classified as a neglected tropical disease [4].

The knowledge on the geographical distribution of the environmental factors for the persistence of the lifecycle is scarce [8, 9]. Studies to improve the knowledge on epidemiological risk factors should be encouraged to enable risk-based sampling. *Echinococcus* notification should always be done at species level in order to discriminate between the more severe alveolar and the cystic echinococcosis [10, 11]. Updated knowledge on the *Echinococcus* parasitism was also discussed for the potential application in immunotherapeutic against parasites and other immune disorders.

2. Transmission

The life cycle of *Echinococcus* species requires a predator-prey relationship between the definitive and intermediate hosts.

E. granulosus is adapted to an environment in which livestock farming plays a central role, completing its cycle through dogs or wild carnivorous animals (as definitive host) and a variety of livestock species, mainly sheep, cattle, pigs, horses, goats, and camels as well as the several wild ungulate species serve as intermediate hosts for the different lineages of the *E. granulosus* species complex [12]. In contrast, several wild rodent species (typically rodents of the families *Arvicolidae* and *Cricetidae*) are the natural intermediate host for *E. multilocularis* [12, 13].

The intermediate hosts become infected through ingestion of eggs in contaminated food or water [12]. The host digestive enzymes dissolve the egg's shell, releasing the oncosphere, which burrows through the host's gut wall and is transported via blood or lymph to the target organ of liver for AE, but mainly liver and lungs, as well other organs for CE [14]. While the life cycle of *E. multilocularis* is completed after a fox or canine consumes a rodent infected with alveolar echincoccosis [8]. Once again adults begin to release a new gravid proglottid, which usually carries some 1500 eggs [15], to be passed to the outside environment with their feces. The adult worms are hermaphroditic. *E. granulosus* becomes prepatent in 32–80 days in the definitive hosts [16], this period varies with the species or strain. While *E. multilocularis* usually becomes prepatent in foxes or dogs in 28–35 days [17], the life cycle of *E. multiloculcaris* is predominantly sylvatic [18].

Humans can serve as an aberrant intermediate host, acquiring the infection by accidental ingestion of eggs, due to handling of infected animals or ingesting contaminated food, vegetable, and water. Except in rare cases, where infected humans are eaten by canines [19], humans are a deadend for *Echinococcus* species, which means that this kind of intermediate host does not allow transmission to the definitive host [20].

Briefly, the disease is spreading when food or water contains the eggs of the parasite, which may be eaten by intermediate animals (such as sheep for *E. granulosus* and rodents for *E. multilocularis*), or due to close contact with an infected definitive animal (carnivorous animals, e.g., dogs, foxes), while the definitive animals, to become infectious, they must eat the organs of an intermediate animal that contains the valid cysts.

3. The parasitism establishment

Generally, selective pressure between host and parasite (parasitism relationship) provides chance for coevolution [21, 22]. A constant adaptation occurs in both populations due to an accumulation of the genetic changes that results in the development of new parasitic strategies and new host defenses [21].

Parasites with complex life cycles often behave differently in their intermediate and definitive hosts [1, 23]. *Echinococcus* species presents strongly affected its intermediate hosts (moose or and small mammals, and rodents) due to high virulence but low virulence in the definitive hosts (such as wolf, fox, or dog). The strong effect makes the intermediate hosts to be more severe sick and easily be captured/hunted by the carnivorous animals [9, 18], thus, benefit parasitic life-cycle and increase transmission dynamics.

The relationship between *Echinococcus* species and their intermediate hosts leads to the necessity for the pathogen to have the virulent alleles to infect the organism and for the host to have the resistant alleles to survive parasitism. Variation in the pathogenicity of strains/species of *Echinococcus* is well known to influence the prognosis in patients with echinococcosis [23]. Increasing epidemiological evidence suggests that certain strains of *E. granulosus* (such as those adapted to horses and pigs) may not be commonly infective to humans [1], and the transmission of parasite strain differs (genetically) geographically and host-adaptively [24]. Therefore, estimates of gene flow between populations in different intermediate hosts or geographic areas can have valuable epidemiological applications [1, 11]. In the genomes of cestodes, considerable gene gain and gene loss associated with the adaptation to parasitism has been found in recent genome parasitic programs [21, 22]. Although, the different morphologies of their metacestode stages caused by *E. multilocularis* and *E. granulosus* are clinically often regarded as "distinctly different entities" [25], they are highly similar concerning gene structure and gene content [22]. Salient differences were so far only observed in the *Echinococcus*-specific apomucin gene family [21]. This is presumably associated with one of the few clear morphological differences between two species of *E. multilocularis* and *E. granulosus*, the thickness of the laminated layer, since the apomucin gene family encodes important components of this structure [26].

4. Interaction between *Echinococcal* parasites and their hosts

During echinococcosis infections (including AE and CE), the distinguishing feature of the host-parasite interaction is that chronic infection coexists with detectable humoral and cellular responses against the parasite [27]. It is well known that the *Echinococcus* species can actively interact with host's both innate and acquired immune systems to maintain their survival with successful evasion from host's immune attacks [28]. The disease spectrum is clearly dependent on the genetic background of the host, as well as on the acquired disturbances of Th1-related immunity [29], such as pregnancy [30], malnutrition [4], severe stress due to work or life [4], coinfection (e.g., HIV) [31, 32], or using immune-suppressing drugs [4, 28]; thus, this kind of circumstances can provide an opportunity to allow the pathogen invading. Human AE appears to be an example of "opportunistic infection", when you make your immunity capability weakness [28, 30]. The genetic constitution of both hosts and pathogens is involved, host genes controlling resistance or susceptibility to infection, genes of the pathogen determining characters such as virulence [23].

In order to establish a successful infection, parasite releases molecules that directly modulate the host immune responses favoring and perpetuating parasite survival in the host [33]. Recent experimental evidence suggests that parasites can not only evade immune responses actively but also exploit the hormonal microenvironment within the host to favor their establishment and growth [34]. Hormonal host parasite cross communication facilitated by the relatively close phylogenetic relationship between *E. multilocularis* and its mammalian hosts, thus appears to be important in the pathology of AE [35]. *E. multilocularis* metacestode metabolic pathway cascades can be activated by host's cell signaling [13, 36], resulting in the larvae development [37]. Conversely, the larval *Echinococcus* can also influence their host immunity response and metabolic signaling mechanisms through the secretion of various molecules [24]. Therefore, immunomodulatory activities of *Echinococcus* and pathological consequences on the host's tissues were attracted by many research concerns for decades [38].

The laminated layer could also play a role similar to that of the placenta at the materno-fetal interface [39]: ensuring parasite growth and infected tissue cell homeostasis while ensuring proper immune tolerance. Tolerance is essential to ensure growth and development of the larval stages of *Echinococcus* species in their hosts [27]. It has been recognized that a series of host-adapted species in the genus *Echinococcus* fits in nicely with observations on host range [1], life cycle, and transmission patterns in areas where echinococcosis is endemic [23]. The ability of hosts to regulate parasites through innate and adaptive immune responses is one of the most important determinants affecting levels of infection, both in the individual and the population [1]. Immunomodulation and, to some extents, immune tolerogenic role have been a great interest of researchers during echinococcosis infection both in human and in animal studies. Many reports have described the worms achieve to switch in the host's response by releasing molecules that share epitopes (and possibly functional activity) with host cytokines [40]. The high relevance for host parasite interaction mechanisms is also found that the presence of evolutionarily conserved signaling systems in *Echinococcus,* such as components of the epidermal growth factor (EGF), fibroblast growth factor (FGF), transforming growth factor ß (TGF-ß), and insulin signal transduction cascades [40, 41], though the signaling systems in animals are also known to be primarily influenced by both factors of the genetic heritage and living environments [42].

The host-derived EGF is known to induce the *Echinococcus* mitogen-activated protein kinase (MAPK) cascade, probably through direct interaction with parasite EGF-receptors [13]. Parasitic components, and not only factors from host origin, were actually acting on hepatocyte metabolic pathways. Recent report indicated that host insulin acts as a stimulant for parasite development within the host liver and that *E. multilocularis* senses the host hormone through an evolutionarily conserved insulin signaling pathway [13, 35].

Although both parasites and hosts benefit from the dynamic balance that grantees parasite-induced damage to hosts at a reasonable level and in turn [42], to some extent, provide parasites nutrients, in some cases of human echinococcosis, spontaneous healing of the disease was observed [20, 27]. Such abortive cases are characterized by calcified parasite lesions suggesting the generation of immune responses which are able to limit parasite growth in humans [27].

5. Disease in animal hosts

A carnivore animal is the definitive host—where the adult worms live in the intestines; and almost any mammal, including humans, can be the intermediate host—where the worms form cysts in various organs for CE but mainly in liver for AE.

5.1. Infection in definitive hosts (mainly implication for dogs)

It is much more difficult to tell when a dog is infected with *Echinococcus* compared to other tapeworms such as *Taenia* or *Dipylidium* [16, 17]. An adult *Echinococcus species* is tiny—only a few millimeters long. Dog infection generally does not show any signs of illness at all even though the hundreds or thousands of tapeworms live in its intestine. Despite the difficult differentiation of the eggs between *Echinococcus* and *Taenia* species under microscopy through fecal examinations [16, 17], the diagnosis of dog infection is an important and useful through dog-copro-DNA assays [16, 17, 43]. So, dog fecal examinations should be performed regularly.

5.2. Infections in intermediate animal hosts

For AE: the primary metacestodes are found in rodent's liver. The germinal membrane of *E. multilocularis* proliferates externally, rather than internally, to form a multilocular structure with many small cysts. These vesicles are usually 1–10 mm in diameter. Hundreds to thousands of protoscolices develop from the germinal membrane in some animal intermediate hosts (small mammals). These multilocular cysts have semisolid matrix and resemble malignant tumors. The center of lesion may be necrotic. The lesion can completely infiltrate an organ, and spread to other organs and tissues nearby. The cysts can also metastasize to distant sites. Although, the tumor-like cysts can kill rodents within a few weeks of infection, this parasite has recently evolved into an experimental model system by use of rodent species to study larval cestode development and associated host-parasite interaction mechanisms.

For CE: the intermediate hosts include a large number of domesticated and wild animals, particularly herbivores. The rate of development varies with the intermediate host and species of parasite, but the cysts usually grow slowly. Their diameter generally increases from less than 1 to 5 cm every year. The parasitic cyst comprises of two walls of an outer laminated membrane and an inner membrane called the germinal layer. All the brood capsules can be produced from the germinal membrane. If the cyst contains protoscolices, it will be named as fertility cyst. Some cysts are sterile, since protoscolices are not produced or killed by bacterial infection. The percentage of sterile cysts varies with the different intermediate host and its susceptibility to a particular strain/species of parasite. The cysts in livestock also seem to be asymptomatic, probably due to the relatively short lifespan of these animals. Because the cyst grows slowly and the symptoms can only appear until its size can effect on adjacent tissues and organs. Occasionally, symptoms have been reported in sheep [5]. But mostly the infected livestock shows poor growth, weakness, and lameness. Therefore, the economic loss assessment modeling due to livestock infections (mainly in sheep) has attracted some extensive attentions in endemic regions and countries worldwide.

6. Disease in humans

Epidemiological studies have demonstrated that the majority of human individuals exposed to infection with *Echinococcus* spp. eggs exhibit resistance to disease as shown by either seroconversion to parasite specific antigens or the presence of "dying out" or "aborted metacestodes" [4]. Seroconversion proving infection, but lack of any lesion indicating the failure of the parasite to establish and further develop within human tissues (mainly in liver) or resistance as shown by the presence of fully calcified lesion [44]; while the developing parasite can be partially controlled by host immunity in those susceptibility individuals where infection leads to disease, as found in the AE and CE patients who experience clinical signs and symptoms approximately 5–15 years after infection [20, 30].

If untreated or uncontrolled, the hyper proliferation of the metacestode due to an impaired immune response could be resulted by immune modulation of host immunity toward energy that can be triggered by parasite metabolites [38], and/or be resulted by additional clinical conditions, such as AIDS or any other reason to induce the immune deficiencies [20, 27, 30]. The disease often starts without symptoms, and this may last for years. The symptoms and signs can occur depend on the lesion location and size for CE. While, AE usually begins in the liver but can spread to other parts of the body.

Cystic echinococcosis (CE) can cause very severe symptoms, if the cyst bursts (e.g., from sudden trauma) or even fatal. The released protoscolices can spread the parasite to other parts of the body to form many new cysts [20].

Alveolar echinocococcis (AE) ranges in size from a sesame seed to a large melon [45]. Although, the mass lesions grow slowly, the tumor-like growth manner tends to invade neighbor organs or tissues, making treatment very difficult [30].

Fibrosis is an important component of the pathophysiology of each disease caused by *Echinococcus* species. However, this role differs markedly in CE and AE. In CE, the rapidly established periparasitic fibrosis surrounding the laminated layer contributes to the unicystic feature of the disease and to limit cyst growth [46]. In AE, the slow fibrogenesis in an extensive and partially unsuccessful periparasitic granuloma does not prevent germinal layer budding.

In the long term, it eventually leads to a dense and irreversible fibrosis, responsible for the main complications of the diseases, such as bile duct, vessel obstruction, and secondary biliary cirrhosis [47–49].

7. Human disease diagnosis

Echinococcal lesions may grow for years, depending on their location, without causing any signs of illness in people [4]. The signs of illness do occur in late stages of diseases, such as abdominal pain and jaundice due to obstruction of bile ducts (in liver), chest pain and difficulty in breathing (in lungs) [4], neurological signs, and seizures (in brain) [30]. Cysts/lesions are sometimes found occasionally when tests are performed for other reasons [4]. Generally, the clinical symptoms and image presentations, e.g., radiographs, ultrasound, CT, or MRI, need to combine the evidences from a blood test for antibodies to the parasite or biopsy for histopathological examination or PCR assay to confirm the diagnosis [4]. Screening individuals living in high-risk areas by ultrasound and serological investigation [44] can catch the infection early and can make treatment much easier and more effective [44].

Therefore, diagnosis requires a combination of tools that involve imaging, histopathology, or nucleic acid detection, and serology. The ultrasound though computer tomography (CT) or magnetic resonance imaging (MRI) may be used commonly. Serology methods for antibodies against the parasite detection can be some certain supplemental tool for imaging/clinical diagnosis. The histopathology or nucleic acid using biopsy after invading methods could provide the final confirmation [4, 20].

8. Management of echinococcosis in human

The growth of larva of *Echinococcus* spp. and the proliferation of the larva are similar to a slow-growing tumor. If the lesion occurs in liver, it can damage liver function. Sometimes, it is difficult to differentiate it from liver cancer because of invasion to biliary and vascular tissue of the liver [50]. Early diagnosis and radical surgery provide the best chance for treatment and cure. Although, treatment of AE is less effective than treatment of CE, the general approach for both types of echinococcosis treatment remains to be surgery with the purpose of complete resection of infected parts of involved organs [4]. Antiparasitic drugs cannot kill cysts if the lesions have already established. However, if untreated, patient survival time is very limited. Therefore, early detection and treatment are important ways to improve patients' survival [4, 20].

Although treatment of cystic echinococcosis by surgery to remove the hydatid cyst was always a risk that the cyst would burst during the procedure, resulting in a very severe, even fatal reaction in the patient to the spilled fluid, drug therapy alone is usually not enough to eliminate cysts, but it can help reduce lesion size and operation risks. More recently, treatment with antiparasitic drugs and drainage of the fluid from the cyst using a needle has been used to treat the disease in certain cases without surgery. Briefly, with proper care, 96–98% of CE patients survive [20].

9. *Echinococcus* species infective risk to humans

The risk of infection with *E. granulosus* or *E. multilocularis* to humans from most pets is very low, but it is higher risks for those residents living in endemic areas. Their work or recreational activities involve direct contact with contaminated water, soil, and their dogs for a long time or life time [10]. Those dogs may allow to roam, hunt, and eat raw tissues from potentially infected animals (e.g., rodents, rabbits, sheep, moose) [8].

The risks for the susceptible of infection with *Echinococcus* spp. can occur in those peoples with immune-compromised conditions (e.g., HIV/AIDS patients, transplant recipients, cancer patients) or with other complications because their immune systems cannot fight infections efficiently [20]. Mostly, ingestion of *Echinococcal* eggs occurred in early ages, if they have chance to contact with contaminated environments, but the disease may appear until they are adults [44].

10. Prevention and control program

Dogs if allowed to enter *Echinococcus*-free areas from potential endemic areas need to be treated with anthelmintic agents (e.g., Praziquantel). Routine inspection of the potential parasitic intermediate host animals before permitting for importing could also prevent the parasite into a country [15].

In endemic areas, dogs should not be allowed to eat the carcasses, particularly the viscera of potential intermediate hosts. Dogs should also be kept from hunting wild rodents and small mammals [6]. Regular examination and treatment of dogs [8] can decrease echinococcosis in domesticated livestock [14].

Prevention of *Echinococcus* species spreading is by treating dogs that may carry the disease and vaccination of sheep. Health education programs focused on echinococcosis and its agents, and improvement of the water sanitation attempt to target poor economic living condition and poor drinking water sources. Educational material should include information about proper disposal of sheep viscera in abattoirs and proximity to dogs and sources of transmission [15].

11. Parasitism perspective applications

11.1. Treatment parasitic infections

In the absence of fully effective antiparasitic chemotherapy for AE and CE, modulation of the host's immune response could be envisaged to fight against the parasite and to prevent the disease and/or its complications such as using IFN-a2a immunological treatment [28] and some parasitic antigens as potential vaccination to prevent disease occurrence such as using Em14-3-3, Em 95, EMY162, and EmTetraspanin [24]. Additionally, current picture on *Echinococcus* signaling systems will be given and the potential to exploit these pathways as targets for antiparasitic chemotherapy [51].

11.2. Using parasite productions for cancer treatment

The presence of Tn antigen in larval and adult tissues of *E. granulosus* was reported [52], this finding is interested in cancer-associated mucin-type because this parasite produced peptides can act on the nonspecific natural killer cell to express cytokines that are effective agents against tumor growth; therefore, the family of Tn antigens might be useful targets for antitumor immunotherapy [41, 53, 54]. These evidences may contribute to the design of tumor vaccines and open new horizons in the use of parasite-derived molecules that can fight against cancer [55, 56].

Cancer vaccination is an important and promising approach in cancer immunotherapy. Obstacles for clinical success may include immune tolerance to TAAs [57], the weak antigenic nature of TAAs, and active immune evasion mechanisms employed by progressing tumors [58]. Vaccination with TAAs coming from evolutionary distant organisms (such as *E. granulosus*) should be useful to override tolerance problems encountered with human TAA-based cancer therapeutic approaches [58].

11.3. Echinococcosis diagnosis

Additionally, the high level of the O-glycosylated Tn antigens generated from larvae of *E. granulosus* are found in the sera of the patients with cystic echinococcosis (CE), providing a pathway that a series of Tn antigens might be sort as a biomarker for this parasitic disease diagnosis, but the hypothesis needs more work to verify the clinical values regarding those antigens [59].

12. Conclusions

Overall, genus *Echinococcus* can be thought an example of successful adaptation to their hosts extensively. Taken advance of recent research outcomes, the parasite immunotherapy for human echinococcosis has been discussed widely by scientific literatures, but importantly, the advanced outcomes may also be interested in terms of using parasites' productions for treatment of other diseases, including cancer.

Acknowledgments

We acknowledge financial support by the National Health and Medical Research Council (NHMRC) of Australia of a NHMRC Project Grant (APP1009539). National Science Foundation of China (NSFC) of the NSFC Project Grants (30960339 and 81460311).

Author details

Shukun Yang[1], Yumin Zhao[2], Don Peter McManus[3] and YuRong Yang[4]*

*Address all correspondence to: yangyurong@hotmail.com

1 Image Diagnosis Department, The First Peoples' Hospital of Yinchuan City, Ningxia Hui Autonomous Region (NHAR), P.R. China

2 Human Pathological Department of Guiling Medical College, Guilin City, Guangxi Province, P.R. China

3 Molecular Parasitology Laboratory, QIMR Berghofer Medical Research Institute, Brisbane, Australia

4 Human Pathology & Immunology Department, Ningxia Medical University, Yinchuan City, Ningxia Hui Autonomous Region (NHAR), P.R. China

References

[1] McManus DP, Thompson RC. Molecular epidemiology of cystic echinococcosis. Parasitology. 2003;**127**(Suppl):S37-S51

[2] Xiao N, Qiu J, Nakao M, Li T, Yang W, Chen X, Schantz PM, Craig PS, Ito A. *Echinococcus shiquicus* n. sp., a taeniid cestode from Tibetan fox and plateau pika in China. International Journal for Parasitology. 2005;**35**:693-701. DOI: 10.1016/j.ijpara.2005.01.003

[3] Hüttner M, Nakao M, Wassermann T, Siefert L, Boomker JD, Dinkel A, Sako Y, Mackenstedt U, Romig T, Ito A. Genetic characterization and phylogenetic position of *Echinococcus felidis* (Cestoda: Taeniidae) from the African lion. International Journal for Parasitology. 2008;**38**:861-868. DOI: 10.1016/j.ijpara.2007.10.013

[4] McManus DP, Gray DJ, Zhang W, Yang Y. Diagnosis, treatment, and management of echinococcosis. British Medical Journal. 2012;**344**:e3866. DOI: 10.1136/bmj.e3866

[5] Carmena D, Cardona GA. Echinococcosis in wild carnivorous species: Epidemiology, genotypic diversity, and implications for veterinary public health. Veterinary Parasitology. 2014;**202**:69-94. DOI: 10.1016/j.vetpar.2014.03.009

[6] Craig PS, McManus DP, Lightowlers MW, Chabalgoity JA, Garcia HH, Gavidia CM, Gilman RH, Gonzalez AE, Lorca M, Naquira C, Nieto A, Schantz PM. Prevention and control of cystic echinococcosis. Lancet Infectious Diseases. 2007;**7**:385-394. DOI: 10.1016/S1473-3099(07)70134-2

[7] Carmena D, Sánchez-Serrano LP, Barbero-Martínez I. *Echinococcus granulosus* infection in Spain. Zoonoses and Public Health. 2008;**55**:156-165. DOI: 10.1111/j.1863-2378.2007.01100.x

[8] Craig PS, Li T, Qiu J, Zhen R, Wang Q, Giraudoux P, Ito A, Heath D, Warnock B, Schantz P, Yang W. Echinococcosis and Tibetan communities. Emerging Infectious Diseases. 2008;**14**:1674-1675. DOI: 10.3201/eid1410.071636

[9] Pleydell DR, Yang YR, Danson FM, Raoul F, Craig PS, McManus DP, Vuitton DA, Wang Q, Giraudoux P. Landscape composition and spatial prediction of alveolar echinococcosis in southern Ningxia, China. PLoS Neglected Tropical Diseases. 2008;**2**:e287. DOI: 10.1371/journal.pntd.0000287

[10] Yang YR, Craig PS, Sun T, Vuitton DA, Giraudoux P, Jones MK, Williams GM, McManus DP. Echinococcosis in Ningxia Hui Autonomous Region, northwest China. Transactions of the Royal Society of Tropical Medicine and Hygiene. 2008;**102**:319-328. DOI: 10.1016/j.trstmh.2008.01.007

[11] Yang YR, Rosenzvit MC, Zhang LH, Zhang JZ, McManus DP. Molecular study of Echinococcus in west-central China. Parasitology. 2005;**131**:547-555. DOI: 10.1017/S0031182005007973

[12] Eckert J, Deplazes P. Biological, epidemiological, and clinical aspects of echinococcosis, a zoonosis of increasing concern. Clinical Microbiology Reviews. 2004;**17**:107-135. DOI: 10.1128/CMR.17.1.107-135.2004

[13] Spiliotis M, Konrad C, Gelmedin V, Tappe D, Brückner S, Mösch HU, Brehm K. Characterisation of EmMPK1, an ERK-like MAP kinase from *Echinococcus multilocularis* which is activated in response to human epidermal growth factor. International Journal for Parasitology. 2006;**36**:1097-1112. DOI: 10.1016/j.ijpara.2006.05.008

[14] Cleary E, Barnes TS, Xu Y, Zhao H, Clements AC, Gray DJ, McManus DP, Atkinson JA, Williams GM, Yang Y. Impact of "Grain to Green" Programme on echinococcosis infection in Ningxia Hui Autonomous Region of China. Veterinary Parasitology. 2014;**205**:523-531. DOI: 10.1016/j.vetpar.2014.08.023

[15] Yang YR, McManus DP, Huang Y, Heath DD. Echinococcus granulosus infection and options for control of cystic echinococcosis in Tibetan communities of Western Sichuan Province, China. PLoS Neglected Tropical Diseases. 2009;**3**:e426. DOI: 10.1371/journal.pntd.0000426

[16] Ni XW, McManus DP, Lou ZZ, Yang JF, Yan HB, Li L, Li HM, Liu QY, Li CH, Shi WG, Fan YL, Liu X, Cai JZ, Lei MT, Fu BQ, Yang YR, Jia WZ. A comparison of loop-mediated isothermal amplification (LAMP) with other surveillance tools for *Echinococcus granulosus* diagnosis in canine definitive hosts. PloS One. 2014;**9**:e100877. DOI: 10.1371/journal.pone.0100877

[17] Ni XW, McManus DP, Yan HB, Yang JF, Lou ZZ, Li HM, Li L, Lei MT, Cai JZ, Fan YL, Li CH, Liu QY, Shi WG, Liu X, Zheng YD, Fu BQ, Yang YR, Jia WZ. Loop-mediated isothermal amplification (LAMP) assay for the identification of *Echinococcus multilocularis* infections in canine definitive hosts. Parasites & Vectors. 2014;**7**:254. DOI: 10.1186/1756-3305-7-254

[18] Yang YR, Liu TX, Bai XL, Boufana B, Craig PS, Nakao M, Ito A, Zhang JZ, Giraudoux P, McManus DP. Natural infection of the ground squirrel (*Spermophilus* spp.) with *Echinococcus granulosus* in China. PLoS Neglected Tropical Diseases. 2009;**3**:e518. DOI: 10.1371/journal.pntd.0000518

[19] Kenny JV, MacCabe RJ. Sero-epidemiology of hydatid disease in the non-intervention area of north-east Turkana. Annals of Tropical Medicine and Parasitology. 1993;**87**: 451-457

[20] Brunetti E, Kern P, Vuitton DA; Writing Panel for the WHO-IWGE. Expert consensus for the diagnosis and treatment of cystic and alveolar echinococcosis in humans. Acta Tropica. 2010;**114**:1-16. DOI: 10.1016/j.actatropica.2009.11.001

[21] Tsai IJ, Zarowiecki M, Holroyd N, Garciarrubio A, Sanchez-Flores A, Brooks KL, Tracey A, Bobes RJ, Fragoso G, Sciutto E, Aslett M, Beasley H, Bennett HM, Cai XP, Camicia F, Clark R, Cucher M, De Silva N, Day TA, Deplazes P, Estrada K, Fernández C, Holland PW, Hou JL, Hu SN, Huckvale T, Hung SS, Kamenetzky L, Keane JA, Kiss F, Koziol U, Lambert O, Liu K, Luo XN, Luo YF, Macchiaroli N, Nichol S, Paps J, Parkinson J, Pouchkina-Stantcheva N, Riddiford N, Rosenzvit M, Salinas G, Wasmuth JD, Zamanian M, Zheng YD; Taenia solium Genome Consortium, Cai JP, Soberón X, Olson PD, Laclette JP, Brehm K, Berriman M. The genomes of four tapeworm species reveal adaptations to parasitism. Nature. 2013;**496**:57-63. DOI: 10.1038/nature12031

[22] Zheng H, Zhang W, Zhang L, Zhang Z, Li J, Lu G, Zhu Y, Wang Y, Huang Y, Liu J, Kang H, Chen J, Wang L, Chen A, Yu S, Gao Z, Jin L, Gu W, Wang Z, Zhao L, Shi B, Wen H, Lin R, Jones MK, Brejova B, Vinar T, Zhao G, McManus DP, Chen Z, Zhou Y, Wang S. The genome of the hydatid tapeworm *Echinococcus granulosus*. Nature Genetics. 2013;**45**:1168-1175. DOI: 10.1038/ng.2757

[23] Thompson, RC and Lymbery AJ, Genetic variability in parasites and host-parasite interactions. Parasitology. 1996;**112**(Suppl):S7-S22

[24] Zhang S, Hüe S, Sène D, Penfornis A, Bresson-Hadni S, Kantelip B, Caillat-Zucman S, Vuitton DA. Expression of major histocompatibility complex class I chain-related molecule A, NKG2D, and transforming growth factor-beta in the liver of humans with alveolar echinococcosis: New actors in the tolerance to parasites? Journal of Infectious Diseases. 2008;**197**:1341-1349. DOI: 10.1086/586709

[25] Stojkovic, M and Junghanss T. Cystic and alveolar echinococcosis. Handbook of Clinical Neurology, 2013;**114**:327-334. DOI: 10.1016/B978-0-444-53490-3.00026-1

[26] Díaz A, Casaravilla C, Allen JE, Sim RB, Ferreira AM. Understanding the laminated layer of larval Echinococcus II: Immunology. Trends in Parasitology. 2011;**27**:264-273. DOI: 10.1016/j.pt.2011.01.008

[27] Vuitton DA, Zhang SL, Yang Y, Godot V, Beurton I, Mantion G, Bresson-Hadni S. Survival strategy of *Echinococcus multilocularis* in the human host. Parasitology International. 2006;**55**(Suppl):S51-S55. DOI: 10.1016/j.parint.2005.11.007

[28] Vuitton, DA and Gottstein B. *Echinococcus multilocularis* and its intermediate host: A model of parasite-host interplay. Journal of Biomedicine & Biotechnology. 2010;**2010**: 923193. DOI: 10.1155/2010/923193

[29] Brehm K *Echinococcus multilocularis* as an experimental model in stem cell research and molecular host-parasite interaction. Parasitology. 2010;**137**:537-555. DOI: 10.1017/S0031182009991727

[30] Yang YR, Vuitton DA, Jones MK, Craig PS, McManus DP. Brain metastasis of alveolar echinococcosis in a hyperendemic focus of *Echinococcus multilocularis* infection. Transactions of the Royal Society of Tropical Medicine and Hygiene. 2005;**99**:937-941. DOI: 10.1016/j.trstmh.2005.04.020

[31] Sailer M, Soelder B, Allerberger F, Zaknun D, Feichtinger H, Gottstein B. *Alveolar echinococcosis* of the liver in a six-year-old girl with acquired immunodeficiency syndrome. Journal of Pediatrics. 1997;**130**:320-323

[32] Ran B, Shao Y, Guo Y, Yimiti Y, Aji T, Jia J, Shayiding P, Jiang T, Cheng L, Li J, McManus DP, Zhang W, Wen H. Surgical treatment of hepatic cystic echinococcosis in patients co-infected with HIV/AIDS. Journal of Helminthology. 2016;**90**:125-128. DOI: 10.1017/S0022149X15000188

[33] Coakley G, Buck AH, Maizels RM. Host parasite communications-messages from helminths for the immune system: Parasite communication and cell-cell interactions. Molecular and Biochemical Parasitology. 2016;**208**:33-40. DOI: 10.1016/j.molbiopara.2016.06.003

[34] Escobedo G, Roberts CW, Carrero JC, Morales-Montor J. Parasite regulation by host hormones: An old mechanism of host exploitation? Trends in Parasitology. 2005;**21**:588-593. DOI: 10.1016/j.pt.2005.09.013

[35] Hemer S, Konrad C, Spiliotis M, Koziol U, Schaack D, Förster S, Gelmedin V, Stadelmann B, Dandekar T, Hemphill A, Brehm K. Host insulin stimulates *Echinococcus multilocularis* insulin signalling pathways and larval development. BMC Biology. 2014;**12**:5. DOI: 10.1186/1741-7007-12-5

[36] Gelmedin V, Caballero-Gamiz R, Brehm K. Characterization and inhibition of a p38-like mitogen-activated protein kinase (MAPK) from *Echinococcus multilocularis*: Antiparasitic activities of p38 MAPK inhibitors. Biochemical Pharmacology. 2008;**76**:1068-1081. DOI: 10.1016/j.bcp.2008.08.020

[37] Brehm K, Spiliotis M, Zavala-Góngora R, Konrad C, Frosch M. The molecular mechanisms of larval cestode development: First steps into an unknown world. Parasitology International. 2006;**55**(Suppl):S15-S21. DOI: 10.1016/j.parint.2005.11.003

[38] Wang J, Zhang C, Wei X, Blagosklonov O, Lv G, Lu X, Mantion G, Vuitton DA, Wen H, Lin R. TGF-beta and TGF-beta/Smad signaling in the interactions between *Echinococcus multilocularis* and its hosts. PloS One. 2013;**8**:e55379. DOI: 10.1371/journal.pone.0055379

[39] Szekeres-Bartho, J. Immunological relationship between the mother and the fetus. International Reviews of Immunology. 2002;**21**(6):471-495

[40] Brehm K, Spiliotis M. The influence of host hormones and cytokines on *Echinococcus multilocularis* signalling and development. Parasite. 2008;**15**:286-290. DOI: 10.1051/parasite/2008153286

[41] Koziol U and Brehm K. Recent advances in Echinococcus genomics and stem cell research. Veterinary Parasitology. 2015;**213**(3-4):92-102. DOI: 10.1016/j.vetpar.2015.07.031

[42] Wang X, Ding J, Guo X, Zheng Y. Current understandings of molecular biology of *Echinococcus multilocularis*, a pathogen for alveolar echinococcosis in humans – A narrative review article. Iranian Journal of Parasitology. 2015;**10**:329-337.

[43] Liu CN, Lou ZZ, Li L, Yan HB, Blair D, Lei MT, Cai JZ, Fan YL, Li JQ, Fu BQ, Yang YR, McManus DP, Jia WZ. Discrimination between *E. granulosus* sensu stricto, *E. multilocularis* and *E. shiquicus* using a Multiplex PCR Assay. PLoS Neglected Tropical Diseases. 2015;**9**:e0004084. DOI: 10.1371/journal.pntd.0004084

[44] Yang YR, Craig PS, Vuitton DA, Williams GM, Sun T, Liu TX, Boufana B, Giraudoux P, Teng J, Li Y, Huang L, Zhang W, Jones MK, McManus DP. Serological prevalence of echinococcosis and risk factors for infection among children in rural communities of southern Ningxia, China. Tropical Medicine & International Health. 2008;**13**:1086-1094. DOI: 10.1111/j.1365-3156.2008.02101.x

[45] Vuitton DA, Benzimidazoles for the treatment of cystic and alveolar echinococcosis: What is the consensus? Expert Review of Anti-Infective Therapy. 2009;**7**(2):145-149. DOI: 10.1586/14787210.7.2.145

[46] Godot V, Harraga S, Deschaseaux M, Bresson-Hadni S, Gottstein B, Emilie D, Vuitton DA. Increased basal production of interleukin-10 by peripheral blood mononuclear cells in human alveolar echinococcosis. European Cytokine Network. 1997;**8**:401-408

[47] Godot V, Harraga S, Beurton I, Deschaseaux M, Sarciron E, Gottstein B, Vuitton DA. Resistance/susceptibility to *Echinococcus multilocularis* infection and cytokine profile in humans. I. Comparison of patients with progressive and abortive lesions. Clinical and Experimental Immunology. 2000;**121**:484-490. DOI: 10.1046/j.1365-2249.2000.01308.x

[48] Reuter S, Buck A, Manfras B, Kratzer W, Seitz HM, Darge K, Reske SN, Kern P. Structured treatment interruption in patients with alveolar echinococcosis. Hepatology. 2004;**39**:509-517. DOI: 10.1002/hep.20078

[49] Konrad C, Kroner A, Spiliotis M, Zavala-Góngora R, Brehm K. Identification and molecular characterisation of a gene encoding a member of the insulin receptor family in *Echinococcus multilocularis*. International Journal for Parasitology. 2003;**33**:301-312

[50] Garcea G, Rajesh A, Dennison AR. Surgical management of cystic lesions in the liver. ANZ Journal of Surgery. 2013;**83**(7-8):E3-E20. DOI: 10.1111/j.1445-2197.2012.06096.x

[51] Brehm K. The role of evolutionarily conserved signalling systems in *Echinococcus multilocularis* development and host-parasite interaction. Medical Microbiology and Immunology. 2010;**199**(3):247-259. DOI: 10.1007/s00430-010-0154-1

[52] Esendagli G, Abbasoglu O. Immune system in cancer and hydatid disease: Cross-reactivity vs. immune modulation. Parasite Immunology. 2015;**37**(8):427-428.DOI: 10.1111/pim.12200

[53] Turhan N, Esendagli G, Ozkayar O, Tunali G, Sokmensuer C, Abbasoglu O. Co-existence of *Echinococcus granulosus* infection and cancer metastasis in the liver correlates with reduced Th1 immune responses. Parasite Immunology. 2015;**37**:16-22. DOI: 10.1111/pim.12152

[54] Yousofi Darani H, Yousefi M, Safari M, Jafari R. Parasites and immunotherapy: With or against? Journal of Parasitic Diseases. 2016;**40**:217-226. DOI: 10.1007/s12639-014-0533-4

[55] Gundogdu SB, Saylam B, Tez M. Cyst hydatid and cancer: The myth continues. Clinical Chemistry and Laboratory Medicine. Published in Association with the European Federation of Clinical Chemistry and Laboratory Medicine (EFLM), 2016. DOI: https://doi.org/10.1515/cclm-2016-0626.

[56] Daneshpour S, Bahadoran M, Hejazi SH, Eskandarian AA, Mahmoudzadeh M, Darani HY. Common antigens between hydatid cyst and cancers. Advanced Biomedical Research. 2016;**5**:9. DOI: 10.4103/2277-9175.175242

[57] Berriel E, Russo S, Monin L, Festari MF, Berois N, Fernández G, Freire T, Osinaga E. Antitumor activity of human hydatid cyst fluid in a murine model of colon cancer. Scientific World Journal. 2013;**2013**:230176. DOI: 10.1155/2013/230176

[58] Noya V, Bay S, Festari MF, García EP, Rodriguez E, Chiale C, Ganneau C, Baleux F, Astrada S, Bollati-Fogolín M, Osinaga E, Freire T. Mucin-like peptides from *Echinococcus granulosus* induce antitumor activity. International Journal of Oncology. 2013;**43**:775-784. DOI: 10.3892/ijo.2013.2000

[59] Alvarez Errico D, Medeiros A, Míguez M, Casaravilla C, Malgor R, Carmona C, Nieto A, Osinaga E. O-glycosylation in Echinococcus granulosus: Identification and characterization of the carcinoma-associated Tn antigen. Experimental Parasitology. 2001;**98**:100-109. DOI: 10.1006/expr.2001.4620

Section 3

Surgical Management of Hydatid Disease

Chapter 3

Surgical Management of Hydatid Disease

Angeliki Vidoura, Mariana Parisidou,
Christina Chatedaki and Dimitris Zacharoulis

Additional information is available at the end of the chapter

http://dx.doi.org/10.5772/intechopen.70136

Abstract

Management of hydatid disease carries a substantial risk of complications and recurrence. The ultimate goal of surgery is to kill the parasites, evacuate the cyst, remove the germinal layer, and obliterate the residual cavity all while preserving the healthy liver tissue. In endemic areas, a conservative approach is preferred. The open surgeries have a substantial risk of complications, such as bile leakage, parasite contamination, and presence of dead spaces, in which an abscess can form. These complications then have to be managed with more radical surgical approaches. The most commonly used surgical approaches are pericystectomy, partial pericystectomy, and even hepatic resection. With the right indications, subadventitial cystectomy has low postoperative complication, mortality, and recurrence. The condition of the cyst and the patient, the general status of the patient and the cyst size, location, and pathology are factors that indicate the optimal surgical approach.

Keywords: echinococcosis, hydatid disease surgical approach, pericystectomy, cystic hepatic echinococcosis, hepatic hydatid cyst, open surgical approach

1. Introduction

Hydatid disease is a global parasitic zoonosis, mostly found in the northern hemisphere, caused by the larval stages of the dog tapeworm *Echinococcus granulosus*. Humans become intermediate hosts through ingestion of the parasite eggs and are infected directly by contact with dogs or indirectly by contaminated food or dirt. The eggs then develop into larvae after crossing the intestinal wall and migrate to the liver, where they form cysts. The liver is the most frequent site for the cystic lesions seen in hydatid disease, followed by the lung and brain. Liver cysts, such as these usually remain asymptomatic and untreated for years until they compress their adjacent organs, form fistulas into them or even rupture into the abdomen. Complete elimination of the parasite with minimum morbidity and mortality is the goal of the surgical treatment. There are three treatment options (**Table 1**): surgery, medical therapy, and interventional procedures. Management of hydatid cysts in the liver typically involves an open surgical approach with meticulous operative site packing and employment of a variety of conservative and radical operative techniques. This chapter reviews the available surgical approaches used to treat cystic echinococcosis of the liver and summarizes the safety and effectiveness of surgical interventions [1].

Pharmaceutical: medical therapy	• Mebendazole • Albendazole • Praziquantel
Percutaneous	• PAIR technique (puncture, aspiration, injection, reaspiration) • Catheterization (percutaneous evacuation, modified catheterization, dilatable multifunction trocar)
Surgical treatment: open or laparoscopic	• Conservative: external drainage, omentoplasty, capitonnage • Radical: subadventitial pericystectomy, (partial) pericystectomy, hepatic resection

Table 1. Treatment options of echinococcal (hydatid) hepatic cysts.

2. Surgical treatment

To date, surgical management remains the treatment of choice for most cases of hydatid hepatic cysts. It is the only method that allows complete eradication of the parasite, treatment or prevention of complications, and evasion of relapse. Indications for surgical management are mentioned in **Table 2** [9].

In general, the physical condition of the patient and the characteristics of the hydatid cyst indicate the necessity of surgical treatment. In cases where surgical treatment is contraindicated, systematic monitoring in combination with drug therapy—with or without minimally invasive, nonsurgical techniques—is the recommended treatment approach (wait and watch). The goals of surgical treatment are mentioned in **Table 3**.

Indications	Contraindications
• Superficial cysts with a high rupture risk	• Multiple cysts
• Large cysts, containing multiple daughter cysts	• Inactive, difficult to access cysts
• Hepatobiliary communication	• Dead cysts
• Compression of neighboring organs (symptomatic)	• Inactive cysts that are partially or totally calcified
• Pus containing, infected echinococcal cyst	• Very small cysts
• Nonhepatic echinococcal cysts (lungs, kidneys, etc.)	• unsuitable patient's condition
• Cysts exerting pressure on adjacent vital organs	

Table 2. Indications for surgical treatment of hydatid echinococcal hepatic cysts.

• Obliteration of the cyst
• Prevention of intraoperative transfer of the parasites
• Treatment of the remaining hepatic parenchyma
• Identification and treatment of possible hepatobiliary communication

Table 3. The goals of surgical treatment of echinococcal (hydatid) hepatic cysts.

Surgical treatment is reserved for complicated cysts, for example, cysts that develop a biliary fistula or perforated cysts and cysts that contain daughter cysts. In addition, it is a treatment of choice for superficial cysts that are smaller than 10 cm or are at high risk of rupture and for patients not suitable for percutaneous treatment. Complete obliteration of the parasite, evacuation of the cyst cavity, elimination of the residual cavity, inactivation of the parasite, and removal of the germinal layer are the main goals of a surgical approach to treating hydatid disease. There are three treatment approaches, and they consist of a conservative or a radical open approach and a laparoscopic approach [6]. Regardless of the technique chosen to treat each patient, it must be noted that medical treatment with benzimidazole prior to any surgery must take place to achieve sterilization of the cyst content and prevent dissemination or anaphylaxis. The operating field must be scrupulously packed in all cases, along with the use of solutions that are capable of eradicating even the protoscolices of the parasite, within the content of the cyst [2]. Some of the scolicidal solutions used in surgical approaches are hypertonic saline, povidone iodine, hydrogen peroxide, iodine, formalin, silver nitrate, and albendazole. These scolicides can be used alone or in combination. Regarding cystic echinococcosis, deep, endoparenchimatic, or rear cysts, close to large vessels, containing multiple daughter cells or calcified cysts must be treated with open surgery. On the other hand, superficial cysts on the anterior side of the liver are more suitably treated with laparoscopic surgery [3].

Surgical options include radical and conservative surgeries. Recurrence and complication rates tend to be higher with conservative surgery as compared to those with radical surgery. The recurrences are usually relative to failure of complete removal of the endocysts and/or their dissemination during the surgery. As in all techniques, the choice of the patients that will be operated on laparoscopically or openly should be made considering the indications. Known advantages of minimally invasive methods, smaller incision, and shorter hospitalization time also take place here. Most common laparoscopic technique used is that of injection evacuation omentoplasty.

2.1. Conservative operations

In conservative procedures, only the parasitic cyst contents are removed, whereas the pericystic membrane is retained and the residual cavity is managed with different techniques such as omentoplasty, capitonnage, or external drainage. The cyst is exposed safely. The pericystic area and operating field are covered with pads soaked with scolicidal agent to prevent the spillage of parasites into the surrounding tissue and peritoneal cavity. The cyst is punctured and aspirated. Before instilling the scolicidal agent, as much fluid as possible is aspirated to prevent dilution of the scolicidal agent. Then, the scolicidal agent is instilled into the cyst cavity and left for approximately 5–15 minutes [4]. Then, the scolicidal agent is aspirated, and the cyst is unroofed. The cyst contents, such as the germinative membrane and daughter cysts, are evacuated. At this point, the cavity should be explored carefully for any gross communication with the biliary tract and for the presence of exogenous cysts embedded in the wall. The next step in conservative treatment is managing the residual cavity. This can be done using various methods such as external drainage, marsupialization, internal drainage, capitonnage, introflexion, and omentoplasty. The Mabit procedure consists of deroofing the cyst and extraction of the parasite with omentoplasty and external drainage of the cyst cavity. The Posadas procedure consists of deroofing of the cyst with capitonnage (the surgical closure of a cyst cavity by applying sutures so as to cause approximation of the opposition surfaces) of the cavity without drainage. During partial pericystectomy, a deeply situated part of cyst wall is left within the liver. Marsupialization is the surgical exteriorization of a cyst by resection of the anterior wall and suture of the cut edges of the remaining cyst to the adjacent edges of the skin, thereby establishing a pouch of what was formally an enclosed cyst. Conservative surgery is easy, safe, and rapid, but has high morbidity and recurrence rates.

2.2. Radical operations

Radical surgery refers to the removal of the cyst along with the pericystic membrane and parasitic contents; it may also include liver resection if indicated. Radical surgical approach aims toward the eradication or elimination of local relapse or complications due to false orbiting. Additionally, it radically deals with the residual cavity, especially in cysts with partial calcification of the wall and biliary communication. There are two methods: the open-cyst method and the closed-cyst method. Radical procedures include: subadventitial cystectomy, (partial) pericystectomy, and hepatic resection. The subadventitial pericystectomy technique is enabled by understanding the surrounding structure of the cyst. The pericyst consists of two layers of different histological origin. Closest to the liver parenchyma is located the subadventitial layer, which is formed by fibrosis and by compression of the Glisson's capsules and hepatic veins. Next up closest to the parasitic cyst is the exocyst layer, which is caused by granulomatous reaction. In between the exocyst and the adventitial layer, there can be found the pericyst and it is the space formed in the in-between that is ideal for smooth detachment [3]. This approach however is not suitable for patients with cysts near the vital vessels or bile ducts. During the pericystectomy procedure, the cyst is dissected along its boundary with healthy liver tissue, blood vessels, and small biliary structures passing through the plane between the normal liver tissue and cyst are clamped and divided. During a hepatic resection operation, the cyst along with the pericyst and in conjunction with normal hepatic parenchyma is removed. Hepatic resection takes longer time to perform and is associated with more blood loss but presents a low rate of cyst recurrence. Pericystectomy and partial pericystectomy are easy to perform and associated with minimal blood loss and operation time. The rate of recurrence of cysts is lower in subadventitial cystectomy and hepatic resection. Subadventitial cystectomy causes less damage to healthy liver tissue than hepatic resection. In any case, treatment aims to one great common goal, that is, the residual cavity must always be treated with excellent care. This is critical to prevent biliary leakage, biliary fistula, and abscess formation. It is in the hands of the surgeon to decide how to go about treating each case separately, depending on the location of the cyst and always aiming towards the safest and most effective method [3]. Radical surgical approaches are associated with a low risk of postoperative complications, fewer relapse cases, long postoperative hospitalization, and low mortality rates; they are all operations with a high difficulty level mostly suitable for highly specialized to the liver surgeons. Radical surgery is superior to conservative surgery with lower morbidity, mortality, and reoccurrence rates [10].

2.3. The use of radiofrequency energy in hydatid disease surgery

The use of radiofrequency under ultrasound guidance allows for very little blood loss and results in minimal coagulation on the liver parenchyma. Ultrasonography (US)-guided RF pericystectomy is recommended specifically for cases where the cyst is not located near the liver helium (**Figures 1** and **2**) [5].

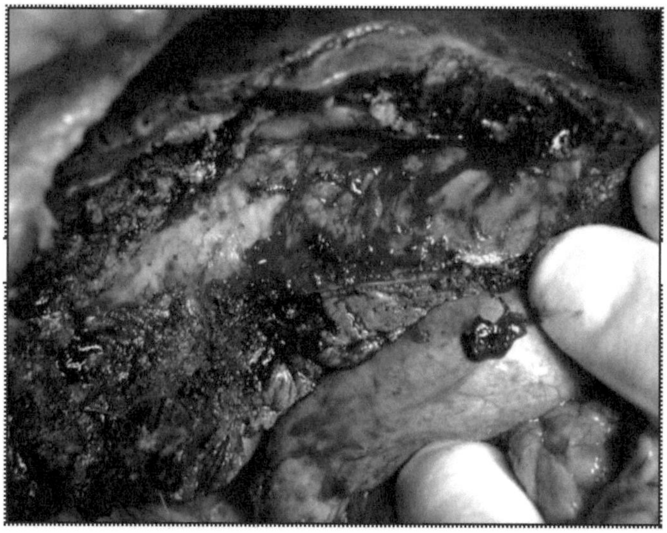

Figure 1. The liver parenchyma is shown with minimal coagulation and hemorrhage, after a radiofrequency assisted closed pericystectomy. (Image kindly supplied by Dr Zacharoulis) [5].

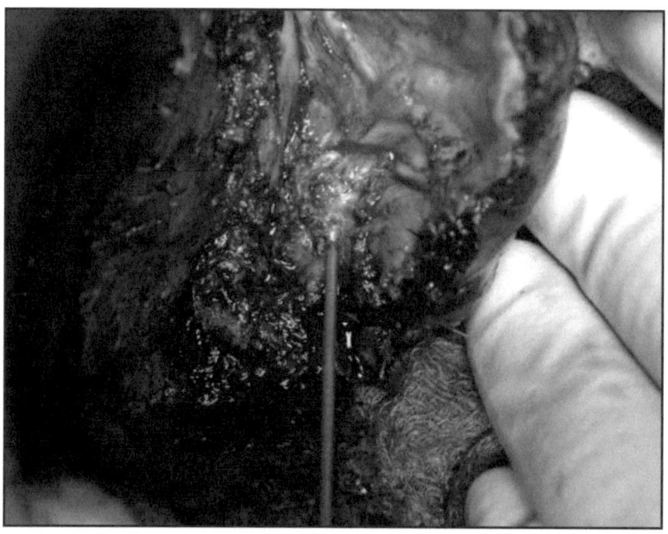

Figure 2. Radiofrequency assisted excision of the pericyst (open pericystectomy). (Image kindly supplied by Dr Zacharoulis) [5].

3. Complication

Potential major complications associated with the surgical treatment of hepatic hydatid cysts include secondary infection; obstructive jaundice due to pressure or rupture into the biliary tree, peritoneum, or an adjacent structure; anaphylaxis, postoperative hemorrhage, bile exudation from the residual cyst cavity, incisional fistula formation, cholangitis, wound infection, sepsis, incisional fistulae; pulmonary complications such as pneumonia and pulmonary embolization; complications of anesthesia; and death. Infection and biliary communication with the cyst (i.e., leakage or rupture with cholestasis) can occur before or after surgical interventions. In the case of intrabiliary rupture either during or after the completion of the operation, treatment can consist of a simple placement of a suture on the orifice, in cases with normal common bile duct caliber and no contamination. In the cases where the common bile duct has an abnormal caliber and the biliary tree is contaminated by cyst contents, firstly the leak must be thoroughly drained and decontaminated and t-tube drainage must be placed, moreover it might even be necessary for a choledochoduodenostomy procedure to be performed. Cases such as these can also be treated endoscopically by sphincterectomy and replacement of the nasobiliary catheter. Another complication or bile leakage which can be symptomatic or cause the formation of a high output biliary fistulae, this can also be managed endoscopically by performing sphincterectomy, nasobiliary drainage, or biliary stenting [7]. Surgical operations except from hepatic resections may leave behind a residual cavity that may easily be mistaken due to imaging techniques for a reoccurrence or any other condition. Recurrence, both local and as secondary echinococcosis, is associated with spillage during removal of the cyst, incomplete removal of the endocyst, and possibly the presence of unnoticed exophytic cyst development. Intraoperative US improves the quality of hepatic surgery [8].

4. Conclusion

In conclusion, hydatid disease remains to be a significant public health problem, and the main treatment goal should be parasite elimination, without recurrence and with minimal morbidity and mortality. Surgical techniques for the treatment of hepatic hydatid cysts range from hepatic resection to simple cyst evacuation and partial pericystectomy. These procedures eventually eradicate the entirety of the parasitic tissue, resulting in complete cure without recurrence. Even though surgical procedures are the golden therapeutic option, an optimal surgical technique is impossible to be decided on since each operation plan is specifically designed to each patient.

Author details

Angeliki Vidoura[1*], Mariana Parisidou[1], Christina Chatedaki[2] and Dimitris Zacharoulis[1]

*Address all correspondence to: angeliki.vid@gmail.com

1 University of Thessaly, Larissa, Greece

2 Department of Microbiology, University Hospital of Larissa, Larissa, Greece

References

[1] Mihmanli M, Idiz UO, Kaya C, Demir U, Bostanci O, Omeroglu S, Bozkurt E. Current status of diagnosis and treatment of hepatic. World Journal of Hepatology. 2016;**8**(28):1169-1181. DOI: 10.4254/wjh.v8.i28.1169

[2] Smego Jr RA, Sebanego P. Treatment options for hepatic cystic echinococcosis. International Journal of Infectious Diseases. 2005;**9**(2):69-76. DOI: 10.1016/j.ijid.2004.08.001

[3] Chen X, Chen X, Shao Y, Zhao J, Li H, Wen H. Clinical outcome and immune follow-up of different surgical approaches for human cyst hydatid disease in liver. The American Society of Tropical Medicine and Hygiene. 2014;**91**(4):801-805. DOI: 10.4269/ajtmh.14-0177

[4] Abdelraouf A, El-Aal AAA, Shoeib EY, Attia SS, Hanafy NA, Hassani M, Shoman S. Clinical and serological outcomes with different surgical approaches for human hepatic hydatidosis. Revista da Sociedade Brasileira de Medicina Tropical. 2015;**48**(5):587-593. DOI: 10.1590/0037-8682-0223-2015

[5] Zacharoulis D, Poultsidis A, Roundas C, Tepetes C. Liver hydatid disease: Radiofrequency-assisted pericystectomy. The Royal College of Surgeons of England. 2006; **88**:499-505. DOI: 10.1308/003588406X116864

[6] Rinaldi F, Brunetti E, Neumayr A, Maestri M, Goblirsch S, Tamarozzi F. Cystic echinococcosis of the liver: A primer for hepatologists. World Journal of Hepatology. 2014;**6**(5):293-305. DOI: 10.4254/wjh.v6.i5.293

[7] Sozuer E, Akyuz M, Akbulut S. Open surgery for hepatic hydatid disease. International Surgery. 2014;**99**(6):764-769. DOI: 10.9738/INTSURG-D-14-00069.1

[8] Graeter T, Ehing F, Oeztuerk S, Mason RA, Haenle MM, Kratzer W, Seufferlein T, Gruener B. Hepatobiliary complications of alveolar echinococcosis: A long-term follow-up study. World Journal of Gastroenterology. 2015;**21**(16):4925-4932. DOI: 10.3748/wjg.v21.i16.4925

[9] Pakala T, Molina M, Wu GY. Hepatic echinococcal cysts: A review. Journal of Clinical and Translational Hepatology. 2016;**4**(1):39-46. DOI: 10.14218/JCTH.2015.00036

[10] Baraket O, Moussa M, Ayed K, Kort B, Bouchoucha S. Predictive factors of morbidity after surgical treatment of hydatid cyst of the liver. Arab Journal of Gastroenterology. 2014;**15**(3-4):119-122. DOI: 10.1016/j.ajg.2014.05.004

Chapter 4

Biliary Complications of Hepatic Hydatid Cyst Surgery and Prevention Methods

Can Konca and Deniz Balcı

Additional information is available at the end of the chapter

http://dx.doi.org/10.5772/intechopen.69031

Abstract

Cystic echinococcosis is still one of the main reasons for liver surgery especially in endemic areas. The most common complication of liver hydatid cyst is cystobiliary communication (CBC). Preoperative or intraoperative diagnosis of CBC is essential for the treatment, since it leads to postoperative bile leakage and fistula formation eventually without intervention. Predictive factors such as cyst size, history of jaundice, and degenerated cysts are described for preoperative evaluation. Further preoperative study can be performed for diagnosis in their presence. At the intraoperative phase, every effort should be performed for diagnosis. There are several methods for the investigation of CBC. When a CBC is found, it is also essential to evaluate the biliary system as well. By this way, postoperative complication rates can be lowered. Biliary leakage and fistula formation are the most common postoperative complication of liver hydatid surgery and they are the main reasons of morbidity and mortality. Their rates can be lowered by knowing how to interfere for the treatment. As a result, every effort should be made to detect and prevent these complications during the evaluation and management of cystic echinococcosis.

Keywords: hydatid cyst, hydatid surgery, bile leakage, bile fistula, biliary complication, prevention, echinococcus

1. Introduction

Cystic echinococcosis (CE) affects liver in approximately 70% of the cases and is still one of the main indications for liver surgery in endemic areas [1]. Reported CE-related mortality rates are between 0.5 and 4%, majority of which are mainly a consequence of the complications [1, 2].

In the past decades, surgery was the only treatment method for hepatic hydatid cysts [3]. With the advancements in medical and percutaneous therapy techniques, surgery is reserved mainly for the complicated hydatid cysts and cysts classified as CE2 or CE3B according to the World Health Organization Informal Working Group on Echinococcosis (WHO-IWGE) classification [1–4].

There are two modalities for surgery: radical and conservative approaches. Pericystectomy (**Figure 1**) and hepatectomy are examples for radical surgery, which aim a complete excision of the cyst and the pericyst [5]. They have lower complication (0–26%) and recurrence (0–3%) rates than the conservative methods [1, 6], but their usage is limited by the anatomic localization and multiplicity of the cysts, since especially in centrally located or bilobular disease, the extent of the surgery exceeds the purpose of the treatment of a benign disease. Also, hepatobiliary surgical expertise and longer operation time are needed for radical surgery, which can be a limitation in endemic regions. By contrast, conservative approaches such as partial pericystectomy (also known as unroofing) with drainage or omentoplasty (**Figure 2**) require less experience and shorter duration of operation. However, their complication and recurrence rates are higher [5]. Simply, they aim to remove the germinal and laminar membrane along with the cystic content and excise the pericystic membrane as much as possible without parenchymal dissection [5]. They have morbidity rates between 6 and 47% and recurrence rates between 4 and 25% [6].

Postoperative bile leakage and fistula formation are a result of cystobiliary communication (CBC) due to intrabiliary rupture (IBR) of the cyst, and this is most common complication of liver surgery for hydatid cyst [7]. Incidence of postoperative bile leakage is between 2.5 and 28.6%. When the postoperative bile leakage is drained externally and persists for more than 10 days, this is called biliary fistula. It is the major cause of morbidity and is encountered in 1–25% of the cases [6, 8]. In the absence of adequate internal or external drainage, bilioma, biliary abscesses, or biliary peritonitis may develop, which can lead to sepsis resulting in serious morbidity and even mortality. Postoperative biliary fistula is the major cause of prolonged hospitalization and complications requiring intervention after hydatid surgery. However, fistulas may close spontaneously in the first postoperative week. It can be classified as "low-flow fistula" if the daily drainage volume is less than 300 ml/day or "high-flow fistula" if more than 300 ml/day [8, 9]. If the fistula persists more than 3 weeks or is a high-flow fistula, then endoscopic or surgical intervention should be considered rather than a conservative approach [8, 10, 11].

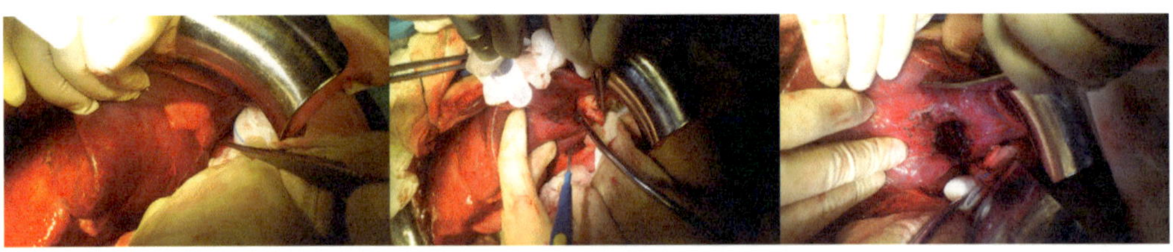

Figure 1. Pericystectomy procedure.

http://dx.doi.org/10.5772/intechopen.69031

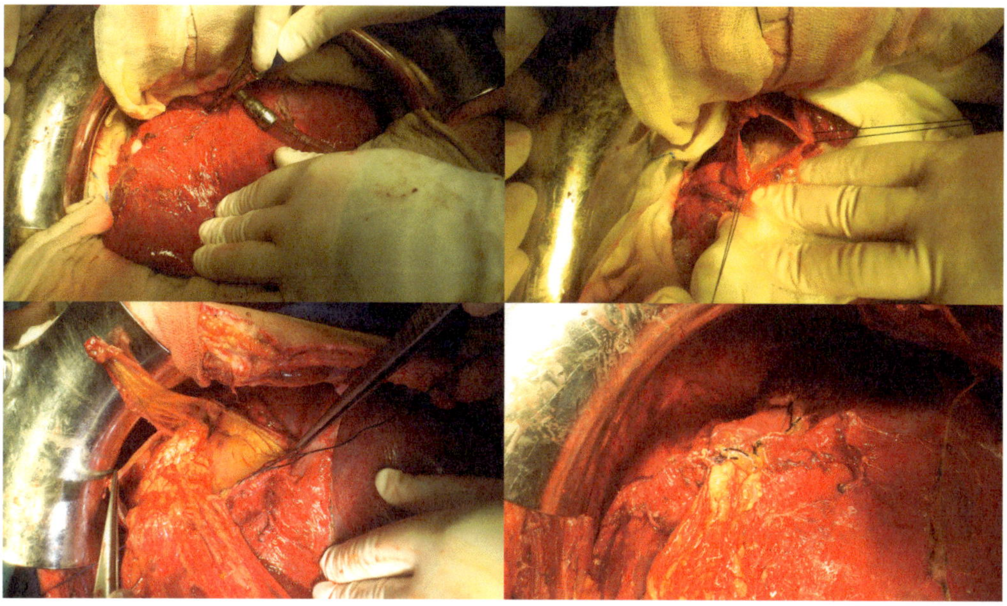

Figure 2. Partial pericystectomy with omentoplasty.

The most common complication of CE is a cystobiliary communication occurring in about 60% of the complicated patients [7]. Two theories have been proposed for pathogenesis: the first is progressive necrosis developing on the wall of biliary duct due to the compression of the hydatid cyst. Such necrosis may lead to a communication between the cyst and the biliary system. The second one suggests that small biliary radicals, which are trapped in the pericystic membrane, become atrophic due to the cystic pressure and rupture eventually [11]. Even though some studies stated communication rates up to 90% during the cysts evolution, the reported incidence of clinical CBC is only 13–37% [8, 11].

There are two types of CBC, **frank** (major, ≥5 mm) and **occult** (minor, <5 mm) CBC [6]. Frank CBC is a wide communication between the cyst and the biliary system. Since intracystic pressure is higher than the biliary pressure, frank CBC allows the cystic contents such as daughter cysts or membrane fragments to enter the biliary system and leads to clinical symptoms like **obstructive jaundice, cholangitis, cyst infection, or anaphylaxis**. Its incidence varies between 3 and 17% in liver hydatid cyst patients [6, 11]. If frank CBC is wider than 5 mm, cystic contents can be seen in the bile ducts during the preoperative evaluation in up to 65% of the patients [11]. Therefore, frank CBC can be diagnosed preoperatively, and treatment can be planned accordingly. By contrast, occult CBC is a smaller communication between the cyst and the biliary radicals. Its incidence varies between 10 and 37% of the patients with liver hydatid cyst [6, 12]. It is usually asymptomatic at the preoperative period, and thus, it is difficult to diagnose. So, careful intraoperative evaluation and postoperative follow-up are needed to overcome the consequences of this morbidity. It is reported that lower postoperative morbidity and bile leakage rates are achieved when the diagnosis is made in the pre- or intraoperative periods [11, 13].

2. Preoperative evaluation

Preoperative evaluation for CBC is essential for liver hydatid surgery, since diagnosis directly affects the treatment plan and the surgical outcome. Diagnosing a frank CBC is easy when a patient presents with symptoms of cholangitis and obstructive jaundice. However, occult CBC is usually asymptomatic and clinical suspicion is essential for its diagnosis. There are few studies investigating the predictive factors for CBC. While Akcan et al. reported that older age, larger cysts, and presence of multiple and bilobar cysts are associated with increased intrabiliary rupture rates, El Nakeeb et al. suggested that only the cyst size (>10 cm) is a significant predictor for CBC, regardless of the type [10, 14]. Because clinical presentation differs between frank and occult CBC, preoperative evaluation will be discussed separately.

2.1. Frank CBC evaluation

Frank CBC can be diagnosed preoperatively. In an unruptured cyst, the intracystic pressure is between 30 and 80 cm H_2O, while the normal intrabiliary pressure is 15 and 20 cm H_2O. When a frank CBC develops, intracystic materials like daughter cysts and membrane fragments, along with the hydatid fluid, enter the biliary ducts as a consequence of the pressure gradient toward the biliary system [8]. Hydatid material in the bile ducts leads to clinical symptoms. Obstructive jaundice can be seen in 57–100% and cholangitis in 20–37% of the patients. Without treatment, both may lead to sepsis and death, with mortality rates as high as 50% [12]. Acute pancreatitis, acute cholecystitis, and, as a late complication, biliary cirrhosis have also been reported [15–17].

In 30–74% of the cases, diagnosis can be made by ultrasonography (US) [11]. Irregular linear echogenic structures without acoustic shadowing in bile duct and a dilated biliary system are ultrasonographic findings in cases with intrabiliary-ruptured frank CBC [6]. The sensitivity of computed tomography (CT) for the diagnosis of frank CBC is 75% [11]. Hydatid materials in the bile ducts or a cystic wall defect due to a frank CBC can be seen via CT. In 75% of the cases, cyst wall discontinuity can be seen as a direct sign of CBC [18]. Magnetic resonance cholangiopancreatography (MRCP) is another alternative and more effective method for the preoperative diagnosis of the suspected cases [18]. For frank CBC diagnosis, MRCP has 92% sensitivity and 83% specificity [11].

There are some clinical predictors described for the presence of frank CBC (**Table 1**) [12]. In our review of 301 cases, our analysis also showed that a high preoperative alkaline phosphatase (ALP), history of cholangitis, and a larger cyst diameter (>10 cm) were significantly more common in patients who developed postoperative biliary fistula (PBF) [19].

History of jaundice
Central location of large cysts >10 cm
Presence of suggestive USG findings
Type IV (Gharbi classification) or CE4 (WHO-IWGE Classification) cyst on USG

Table 1. Clinical predictors of frank CBC.

In cases of clinical suspicion and presence of predictive factors, further studies can be planned such as MRCP or endoscopic retrograde cholangiopancreatography (ERCP). Because MRCP is a noninvasive test, it can be used as a primary method for the diagnosis. After confirmation of CBC diagnosis, ERCP can also be used for treatment [20].

ERCP can be used for both diagnostic and therapeutic purposes. It has 86–100% diagnostic sensitivity for frank CBC. It serves for (i) the treatment of acute conditions to defer for elective surgery, (ii) decreasing the postoperative complication rates and achieving shorter post-operative hospitalization time, and (iii) evacuation of biliary and cystic hydatid contents [20]. ERCP with endoscopic sphincterotomy (ES) is the first line of treatment for patients presenting with jaundice or findings of IBR [11]. In case of documented CBC, it helps with planning the elective surgery and prevention of intraoperative common bile duct exploration during the operation [10–12]. Additionally, lower postoperative biliary fistula rates were reported with preoperative ERCP with ES [11]. Performing ERCP with ES prior to surgery decreases the risk from 11.1 to 7.6% for postoperative biliary fistula [21]. It was also reported that 25% of the patients with frank CBC have been cured with ERCP without the need for further surgery [20]. In addition to ES, extraction with balloon or basket catheter, nasobiliary drainage, and biliary stenting can be used as therapeutic tools during ERCP [20].

2.2. Occult CBC evaluation

Occult CBC is hard to diagnose preoperatively since a small communication usually cannot be seen on radiologic studies [12, 22, 23]. Most of the cases are asymptomatic until surgery or postoperative period when it presents as bile leakage and fistula. The flow gradient of contents is toward the biliary system in an unruptured cyst. As a result, small biliary radicals are compressed with the pressure and remain silent until the gradient is reversed. The median intracystic pressure is around 25 mm Hg (range, 5–55 mm Hg) and there is a positive correlation between cyst size and pressure in viable cysts. Manometric studies indicate that the sphincter of Oddi pressure (basal 10 mmHg, peak 124 mmHg) is higher than the normal common bile duct pressure (10 mmHg). According to the LaPlace Law, the expansion of the cyst due to increased intracystic pressure results in an increased cyst diameter, which causes increased tension on the cyst wall containing the neighboring bile ducts. The pressure dynamics arising from higher intracystic pressures than the resting bile duct pressure may explain how the cyst communicates with the biliary system as the pericyst becomes thinner and thinner, eventually eroding into the bile ducts and leading to the development of an IBR [19]. During an operation with conservative approach, bile staining of the cystic content during first aspiration cannot be seen in most cases. Once the gradient is reversed with aspiration and evacuation of the cystic content, bile leakage begins [8]. So, the principal evaluation of occult CBC must be undertaken during surgery. Even with an attempt to control a detected BF intraoperatively, there might be a significant failure rate if that was used as the only method to control the cyst-biliary communication [19].

However, there are some clinical predictors described for the presence of occult CBC (**Table 2**) [8, 12]. Taking these predictors into consideration, a clinical suspicion can further lead to evaluation for an occult CBC. However, unlike frank CBC, diagnostic sensitivity of MRCP and ERCP is low [12]. In cases with high suspicion, preoperative ERCP with ES can be done to decrease the postoperative leakage rate and to determine the biliary anatomy [20]. Yet, this is not a standard therapeutic modality.

A diagnostic and therapeutic algorithm for preoperative evaluation of CBC can be seen in **Figure 3**.

History of nausea and vomiting
ALP level >144 U/L
gamma-glutamyltransferase (GGT) level >34.5 U/L
Total bilirubin level >0.8 mg/dL
Direct bilirubin level >0.4 mg/dL
Eosinophil rate >0.09
Cyst diameter >8.5 cm
Multilocular cysts (Gharbi type III)
Degenerate cysts (Gharbi type IV or WHO-IWGE CE4)

*The data in this table are derived from different studies having common and uncommon predictive parameters and among similar parameters, ones with the lowest cut-offs were selected to aim for the widest patient range [8, 12].

Table 2. Clinical predictors of occult CBC*.

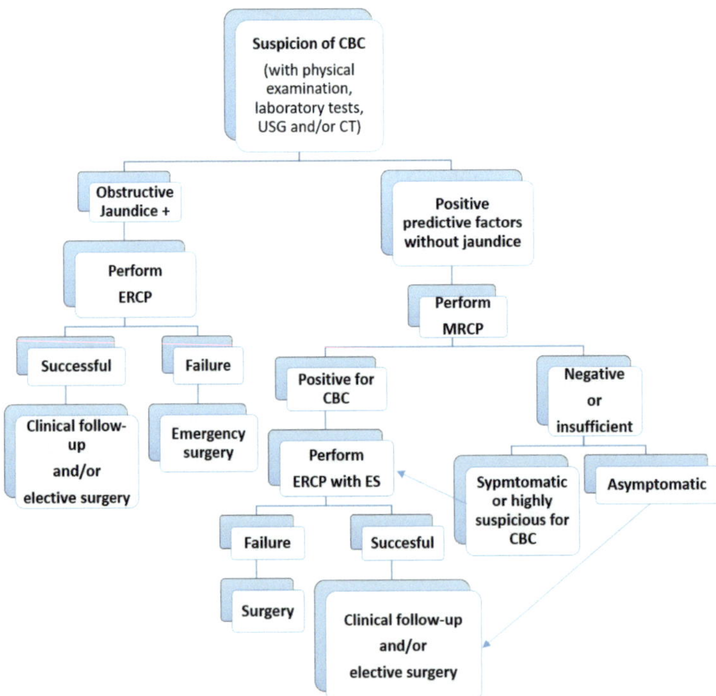

Figure 3. Diagnostic and therapeutic algorithm for preoperative evaluation of CBC.

http://dx.doi.org/10.5772/intechopen.69031

3. Operative decision making

Radical surgical techniques should be undertaken whenever feasible because of their lower postoperative morbidity and recurrence rates [5, 8, 11]. In the last decade, major liver surgery became much more safer with very low morbidity and mortality rates. The decision making is usually complex with various factors interplaying different roles. Patient-related factors with general condition and comorbidities, liver parenchymal quality (steatosis, age, diabetes, etc.), and center expertise are leading factors. On the other hand, these factors, taken together, may pose a higher risk for a benign disease unless complicated [11]. As a result, conservative approaches are still the most common method applied, especially in the endemic regions [8]. Among all the conservative methods, partial cystectomy with omentoplasty has the lowest reported postoperative leakage rate [1, 24]. In our center, we favor anatomical liver resections whenever feasible, especially in patients with frank CBC.

4. Intraoperative evaluation

Frank CBC is usually easy to diagnose intraoperatively. The communication should be sutured whenever feasible. If it is diagnosed with MRCP or ERCP preoperatively, it is essential to understand the type and anatomical location of the communication of the duct with the cyst. If the frank communication is related with the primary or secondary biliary pedicules, suture closure of the communication could lead to biliary obstruction for distal branches [12]. In such cases, conversion to radical surgery, biliary drainage procedures like t-tube drainage or choledochoduodenostomy or postoperative ERCP and ES with or without biliary stenting/nasobiliary drainage should be considered [11]. In patients with frank CBC without preoperative evaluation, cholangiography or choledochoscopy can be performed before and after the evacuation of hydatid material in bile ducts. After that, placing a t-tube and closure over t-tube or decompression through cystic duct can be preferred [8, 11]. It is reported that when a communication is wider than 5 mm, hydatid material in biliary system can be seen in 65% of the cases [25]. For that reason, an intraoperative cholangiography via the communication, cystic duct, or common bile duct can be done in patients without preoperative ERCP [12].

Careful evaluation should be done to diagnose occult CBC. At the first aspiration of the hydatid cyst fluid, bile staining should be checked. If the fluid is positive for bile, a surgeon should avoid using scolicidal agents to prevent sclerosing cholangitis [2, 6, 11]. After evacuation of the hydatid material in the cyst cavity, careful inspection for bile leakage should be done inside the cavity. Using a coloring scolicidal agent like povidone iodine can be a handicap for this purpose [8]. On the other hand, using a non-coloring scolocidal agent like hypertonic saline or chlorhexidine may increase diagnostic accuracy. If a communication is found, it should be sutured [11].

Surgical telescopes with 2.5 × or 3.5 × magnification can enhance the quality of inspection. In cases of negative inspection for bile leakage, there are several methods for additional evaluation. The simplest method is filling the cavity with gauze [8]. In addition, manual clamping of the main bile duct can provoke bile staining through the communication by increasing intrabiliary pressure. When discovered, occult CBCs should also be sutured. Another method described especially for large and multilobar cysts, which can be at difficult locations for inspection, is using a videotelescope [26]. The rotation and magnification abilities of the videotelescope facilitate a more precise diagnosis, especially in multilobar and deep localized cavities. Endoscopic instruments can also be used for suturation of unreachable communications [26].

When bile staining is present but the communication cannot be localized, there are two options: external drainage from cavity can be performed and postoperative ERCP with ES can be scheduled or, as a more invasive option, methylene blue or air injection with or without intraoperative cholangiography can be performed [11, 12]. In such cases, cholangiography can be performed via cystic duct or main bile duct [12]. A cholecystectomy is needed to perform a transcystic cholangiography. If the patient has cholelithiasis or the gallbladder wall constitutes the cyst wall, then transcystic approach should be preferred. Otherwise, cholangiography through the main duct with a thin-needled syringe—like insulin syringe—should be done. Separately, or in addition to cholangiography, methylene blue or air injection through cholangiography access should be done for detecting the localization of the communication [11, 12, 27]. With methylene blue injection, covering of the cavity with gauze technique can be used for localization. If air injection is preferred, filling the cavity with saline should be done. Next, air bubbles in the cavity must be checked for the presence of a communication.

If a frank or occult CBC has been detected intraoperatively and the patient has not been evaluated preoperatively with MRCP or ERCP, cholangiography should be performed for the presence of hydatid material in the biliary system. In cases with hydatid material, choledochotomy should be done and after evacuation of the hydatid material, t-tube drainage should be performed for further access and evaluation. In cases of biliary stricture, choledochoduodenostomy may be preferred. Intraoperative ERCP can be a less invasive approach in available centers [14, 20].

In all cases that underwent conservative hydatid liver surgery, continuous suturation of pericystectomy line can be used to eliminate the risk of leakage from biliary radicals at pericystic wall and an external drainage catheter should be placed at the entrance or in the cavity to avoid the risk of uncontrolled postoperative biliary leakage and biliary peritonitis.

In some series, fibrin sealant usage to prevent postoperative biliary leakage is used, but controversial results have been reported. Therefore, efficacy of fibrin sealant is still questionable [5, 9].

5. Postoperative evaluation

A close follow-up should be done at the postoperative period for complications. In acute conditions, necessary interventions should be planned promptly. Emergency laparotomy is indicated if the patient has biliary peritonitis. Peritoneal irrigation, correction of leakage by suturation or more radical methods as needed and maintaining an adequate external drainage should be performed accordingly. If bile leakage persists after the operation, ERCP with ES and biliary stenting should be considered [20].

In cases of postoperative jaundice, first therapeutic modality should be ERCP with ES and evacuation of the hydatid contents within the bile ducts [20]. If ERCP fails, then bile duct exploration with t-tube drainage or choledochoduodenostomy should be considered.

Biliomas should be evaluated with percutaneous drainage first. When biliary leakage persists, then ERCP with ES should be scheduled [20].

The most common postoperative complication of hydatid liver surgery is bile leakage and fistula formation as mentioned before. In such cases, every effort should be made at the pre-operative and intraoperative period to decrease its rates. When postoperative bile fistula is present, it is essential to determine the flow rate of fistula. In low-flow fistulas (flow rate of <300 ml/day), conservative follow-up for 3 weeks is appropriate since most of low-flow fistulas close spontaneously in this period [8, 9]. If the fistula persists after 3 weeks, then ERCP

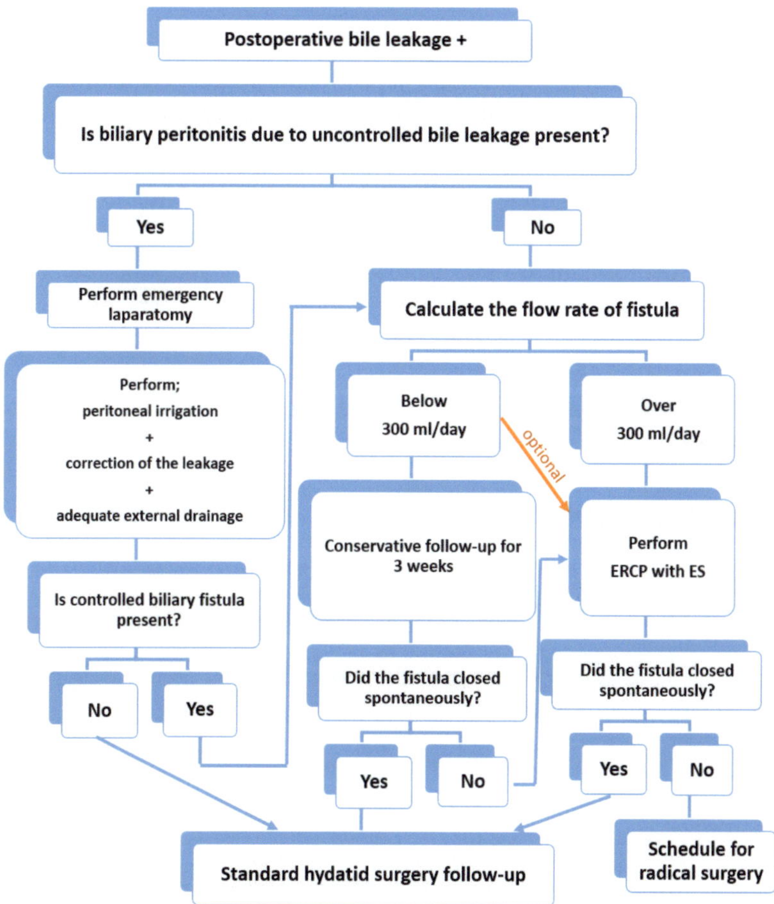

Figure 4. Therapeutic algorithm for postoperative bile leakage.

with ES should be planned [8, 10, 11]. In high-flow fistulas (>300 ml/day), spontaneous closure of the fistula is unlikely; thus, ERCP with ES should be performed without delay [8, 20]. The success rate of ERCP is very high (90%) [11]. Most of the fistulas close in the first week after ERCP [8]. Spontaneous closure of a fistula from a calcified cyst wall is usually unexpected [2]. In our series, PBF occurred in 46 (16%) patients, despite preoperative and operative efforts to prevent this complication. The fistula closed spontaneously in only 12 (26%) of the patients with PBF without further intervention, confirming that patients with PBF often have a complicated postoperative course, requiring multiple endoscopic and other interventional procedures with serious morbidity and mortality [19].

In a small group of patients in whom all interventions fail, as repeated ERCP and stenting, radical surgery could be an alternative for the correction of the leakage [6, 28]. A therapeutic algorithm for postoperative bile leakage evaluation is offered in **Figure 4**.

6. Conclusion

Hydatid liver surgery is still one of the main indications for liver surgery in endemic regions. It is hard to refer all patients to an experienced hepatobiliary surgery center due to high volume of disease in those regions. As a result, conservative methods are still preferred therapeutic modalities for many surgeons.

Cystobiliary communication is the most common complication of hydatid liver disease. Without appropriate evaluation and intervention, this will eventually lead to postoperative bile leakage and fistula formation, a major cause of morbidity and mortality. By that means, every effort should be made to detect and prevent these complications during the evaluation and management of cystic echinococcosis liver disease.

Author details

Can Konca[1] and Deniz Balcı[2*]

*Address all correspondence to: denizbalci1@yahoo.com

1 Department of General Surgery, Ankara University School of Medicine, Ankara, Turkey

2 Department of General Surgery and Transplantation Division of Hepatopancreatobiliary Surgery, Ankara University School of Medicine, Ankara, Turkey

References

[1] Mihmanli M, Idiz UO, Kaya C, Demir U, Bostanci O, Omeroglu S, Bozkurt E. Current status of diagnosis and treatment of hepatic echinococcosis. World Journal of Hepatology. 2016;**8**(28):1169-1181

[2] Brunetti E, Kern P, Vuitton DA, Writing Panel for the WHO-IWGE. Expert consensus for the diagnosis and treatment of cystic and alveolar echinococcosis in humans. Acta Tropica. 2010;**114**(1):1-16

[3] Junghanss T, da Silva AM, Horton J, Chiodini PL, Brunetti E. Clinical management of cystic echinococcosis: State of the art, problems, and perspectives. American Journal of Tropical Medicine and Hygiene. 2008;**79**(3):301-311

[4] Guidelines for treatment of cystic and alveolar echinococcosis in humans. WHO Informal Working Group on Echinococcosis. Bulletin of the World Health Organization. 1996;**74**(3):231-242

[5] Gomez IGC, Lopez-Andujar R, Belda Ibanez T, Ramia Angel JM Moya Herraiz A, Orbis Castellanos F, Pareja Ibars E, San Juan Rodriguez F. Review of the treatment of liver hydatid cysts. World Journal of Gastroenterology. 2015;**21**(1):124-131

[6] Sozuer E, Akyuz M, Akbulut S. Open surgery for hepatic hydatid disease. International Surgery. 2014;**99**(6):764-769

[7] Chautems R, Buhler LH, Gold B, Giostra E, Poletti P, Chilcott M, Morel P, Mentha G. Surgical management and long-term outcome of complicated liver hydatid cysts caused by *Echinococcus granulosus*. Surgery. 2005;**137**(3):312-316

[8] Demircan O, Baymus M, Seydaoglu G, Akinoglu A, Sakman G. Occult cystobiliary communication presenting as postoperative biliary leakage after hydatid liver surgery: Are there significant preoperative clinical predictors? Canadian Journal of Surgery. 2006;**49**(3):177-184

[9] Atahan K, Kupeli H, Deniz M, Gur S, Cokmez A, Tarcan E. Can occult cystobiliary fistulas in hepatic hydatid disease be predicted before surgery? International Journal of Medical Sciences. 2011;**8**(4):315-320

[10] El Nakeeb A, Salem A, El Sorogy M, Mahdy Y, Ellatif MA, Moneer A, Said R, El Ghawalby A, Ezzat H. Cystobiliary communication in hepatic hydatid cyst: Predictors and outcome. The Turkish Journal of Gastroenterology: The Official Journal of Turkish Society of Gastroenterology. 2017;**28**:125-130

[11] Ramia JM, Figueras J, De la Plaza R, Garcia-Parreno J. Cysto-biliary communication in liver hydatidosis. Langenbeck's Archives of Surgery. 2012;**397**(6):881-887

[12] Atli M, Kama NA, Yuksek YN, Doganay M, Gozalan U, Kologlu M, Daglar G. Intrabiliary rupture of a hepatic hydatid cyst: Associated clinical factors and proper management. Archives of Surgery. 2001;**136**(11):1249-1255

[13] Prousalidis J, Kosmidis C, Kapoutzis K, Fachantidis E, Harlaftis N, Aletras H. Intrabiliary rupture of hydatid cysts of the liver. The American Journal of Surgery. 2009;**197**(2):193-198

[14] Akcan A, Sozuer E, Akyildiz H, Ozturk A, Atalay A, Yilmaz Z. Predisposing factors and surgical outcome of complicated liver hydatid cysts. World Journal of Gastroenterology. 2010;**16**(24):3040-3048

[15] Kattan YB. Intrabiliary rupture of hydatid cyst of the liver. Annals of the Royal College of Surgeons of England. 1977;**59**(2):108-114

[16] Saez-Royuela F, Yuguero L, Lopez-Morante A, Perez-Alvarez JC, Martin-Lorente JL, Ojeda C. Acute pancreatitis caused by hydatid membranes in the biliary tract: Treatment with endoscopic sphincterotomy. Gastrointestinal Endoscopy. 1999;**49**(6):793-796

[17] Abou-Khalil S, Smith BM, MacLean JD, Poenaru D, Fried GM, Bret P, Barkun AN. Acute cholecystitis and cholangitis caused by *Echinococcus granulosus*. The American Journal of Gastroenterology. 1996;**91**(4):805-807

[18] Ormeci N, Kir M, Coban S, Emrehan Tuzun A, Ekiz F, Erdem H, Palabiyikoglu M, Dokmeci A. The usefulness of endoscopic retrograde cholangiopancreatography and (99m)Tc-labeled albumin macroaggregates in diagnosing hydatid disease fistulae. Digestive Diseases and Sciences. 2007;**52**(6):1410-1414

[19] Zeybek N, Dede H, Balci D, Coskun AK, Ozerhan IH, Peker S, Peker Y. Biliary fistula after treatment for hydatid disease of the liver: When to intervene. World Journal of Gastroenterology. 2013;**19**(3):355-361

[20] Dolay K, Akbulut S. Role of endoscopic retrograde cholangiopancreatography in the management of hepatic hydatid disease. World Journal of Gastroenterology. 2014;**20**(41): 15253-15261

[21] Galati G, Sterpetti AV, Caputo M, Adduci M, Lucandri G, Brozzetti S, Bolognese A, Cavallaro A. Endoscopic retrograde cholangiography for intrabiliary rupture of hydatid cyst. The American Journal of Surgery. 2006;**191**(2):206-210

[22] Ozaslan E, Bayraktar Y. Endoscopic therapy in the management of hepatobiliary hydatid disease. Journal of Clinical Gastroenterology. 2002;**35**(2):160-174

[23] Spiliadis C, Georgopoulos S, Dailianas A, Konstantinidis A, Rimikis M, Skandalis N. The use of ERCP in the study of patients with hepatic echinococcosis before and after surgical intervention. Gastrointestinal Endoscopy. 1996;**43**(6):575-579

[24] Mentes A, Yuzer Y, Ozbal O, Coker A, Ilter T, Musoglu A. Omentoplasty versus introflexion for hydatid liver cysts. Journal of the Royal College of Surgeons of Edinburgh. 1993;**38**(2):82-85

[25] Zaouche A, Haouet K, Jouini M, El Hachaichi A, Dziri C. Management of liver hydatid cysts with a large biliocystic fistula: Multicenter retrospective study. Tunisian Surgical Association. World Journal of Surgery. 2001;**25**(1):28-39

[26] Ozmen MM, Coskun F. New technique for finding the ruptured bile duct into the liver cysts: Scope in the cave technique. Surgical Laparoscopy, Endoscopy & Percutaneous Techniques. 2002;**12**(3):187-189

[27] Kayaalp C, Sengul N, Akoglu M. Importance of cyst content in hydatid liver surgery. Archives of Surgery. 2002;**137**(2):159-163

[28] Akcakaya A, Sahin M, Karakelleoglu A, Okan I. Endoscopic stenting for selected cases of biliary fistula after hepatic hydatid surgery. Surgical Endoscopy and Other Interventional Techniques. 2006;**20**(9):1415-1418

Section 4

New Horizons for Medical Treatment of Echinococcosis

Chapter 5

Medical Treatment of *Echinococcus multilocularis* and New Horizons for Drug Discovery: Characterization of Mitochondrial Complex II as a Potential Drug Target

Shigehiro Enkai, Kimitoshi Sakamoto, Miho Kaneko, Hirokazu Kouguchi, Takao Irie, Kinpei Yagi, Yuka Ishida, Jun Matsumoto, Yuzaburo Oku, Ken Katakura, Osamu Fujita, Tomoyoshi Nozaki and Kiyoshi Kita

Additional information is available at the end of the chapter

http://dx.doi.org/10.5772/intechopen.68565

Abstract

As an efficient drug for alveolar echinococcosis (AE) is still not available, new chemotherapy targets are necessary. The mitochondrial respiratory chain may be a good drug candidate because parasite respiratory chains are quite different from those of mammalian hosts. For example, *Ascaris suum* possesses an NADH-fumarate reductase system (fumarate respiration) that is highly adapted to anaerobic environments such as the small intestine. It is composed of mitochondrial complex I (NADH-ubiquinone reductase), complex II (succinate-ubiquinone reductase), and rhodoquinone. We previously demonstrated that fumarate respiration is also essential in *E. multilocularis*. Quinazoline, a complex I inhibitor, inhibited growth of *E. multilocularis* larvae in vitro. These results indicate that fumarate respiration could be a target for *E. multilocularis* therapy. In the current chapter, we focused on complex II, which is another component of this system, because quinazoline exhibited strong toxicity to mammalian mitochondria. We evaluated the molecular and biochemical characterization of *E. multilocularis* complex II as a potential drug target. In addition, we found that ascofuranone, a trypanosome cyanide-insensitive alternative oxidase inhibitor, inhibited *E. multilocularis* complex II at the nanomolar order. Our findings demonstrate the potential development of targeted therapy against *Echinococcus* complex II.

Keywords: *Echinococcus multilocularis*, drug discovery, fumarate respiration, mitochondrial complex II, ascofuranone

1. Treatment and prevention of echinococcosis

1.1. Treatment of alveolar echinococcosis

Echinococcosis is a zoonosis caused by adult or larval stage *Echinococcus*, tiny cestode parasites in the family *Taeniidae*. The two major species of medical and public health importance are *Echinococcus granulosus* and *E. multilocularis*, which cause cystic echinococcosis (CE) and alveolar echinococcosis (AE), respectively. This chapter describes the main objective of AE therapy, which is more difficult to treat than CE. Treatment for CE generally includes albendazole, surgery, and puncture, aspiration, injection, and reaspiration (PAIR) therapy, or a combination thereof, according to the World Health Organization diagnostic classification [1, 2]. The cure rate of PAIR therapy is especially high, at 97% for cysts exceeding 5 cm in size [3, 4]. However, PAIR therapy has not been adopted for AE. In surgical treatment of AE, radical resection is required for hepatic lesions. Conservative and palliative surgery are not recommended since they have no advantage over chemotherapy [5]. Liver transplantation is a therapeutic option for patients unsuitable for radical surgery with hepatic failure. Extrahepatic spread of AE in liver transplant recipients may lead to a risk of relapse due to the use of immunosuppressive agents after surgery [6, 7]. In addition, it is not easy to perform liver transplantation in developing countries without advanced medical equipment and high health care costs. As radical surgery for advanced AE is more difficult than that for CE, chemotherapy plays a key role in treatment of AE. Albendazole, a benzimidazole anthelmintic, is primarily used in chemotherapy for AE. The 15-year survival of albendazole treatment is 53–80% in patients not treated by surgery, according to the condition of cysts [3, 8, 9]. Furthermore, two-thirds of patients experienced one or more side effects of albendazole, and the development of major side effects led to permanent discontinuation of albendazole in 3.8% of patients [10]. Praziquantel, which is expected to have a synergistic effect with albendazole, is insufficient for AE [11]. Although in vivo studies have evaluated the effectiveness of a calcium channel blocker, thymol, and novel compounds are reported as new chemotherapy, they have only a limited effect on AE [12–14]. A recent report revealed that nitazoxanide, an anticipated promising drug, had no effect on treatment of AE [15]. These findings emphasize the difficulty in developing an effective drug for AE. Additionally, there are no other treatment options for patients in whom albendazole chemotherapy failed and who have no indications for liver transplantation.

1.2. Current status of the development of a vaccine against echinococcosis

Vaccine targets for echinococcosis are either intermediate or definitive hosts or both. EG95 was identified as a candidate vaccine antigen for intermediate hosts of *E. granulosus* in 1998 [16, 17]. As intermediate hosts of CE are livestock, such as sheep, goat, and cattle, vaccination of intermediate hosts of CE would presumably lead to the reduction of economic loss and the effective control of CE in the life cycle. In a pilot field trial of the EG95 vaccine, vaccine introduction in a sheep farm led to a statistically significant reduction in the number and size of hydatid cysts compared to the control area where the vaccine was not applied. The prevalence of infection in the vaccinated area was reduced by 62% compared to the control area [18].

The gene product of *E. multilocularis*, EM95, is homologous to EG95 [19]. Mice immunized with the EM95 recombinant protein following challenge infection showed a significantly decreased number of cysts compared with control mice [19]. Furthermore, EMY162 antigen, which is also homologous to EG95, was identified in 2007 [20, 21]. Several candidate vaccine antigens based on homology to EM95 or EMY162 were subsequently reported [22, 23]. In addition, a transmembrane protein, tetraspanin (TSP), was identified as the antigen protein of an AE vaccine [24]. Protective effects of recombinant TSP against AE have been reported [25, 26]. However, it is difficult to apply a vaccination strategy to wild mice, which are the main intermediate hosts of AE. Although human AE is a serious parasitic disease, there has been little progress on application of these vaccines to humans since safety standards are exceptionally high.

Development of a vaccine for the definitive host dog is important because such a vaccine might contribute to a considerable reduction of human CE and AE in endemic areas. However, no effective vaccine candidate has been identified despite various trials. Although some oral recombinant vaccines showed high levels of protection against *E. granulosus* in dogs [27–29], these reports have been criticized in terms of their statistical analyses [30]. However, mucosal immunization with a parasite surface antigen, with cholera toxin subunit B as a carrier molecule, induced a protective response to *E. multilocularis* infection in dogs [31]. Immunized dogs infected five times with *E. multilocularis* remained capable of excluding adult worms after a 6-month interval [32, 33]. These results suggest the potential effectiveness of the mucosal vaccine against *E. multilocularis* in definitive hosts.

2. Mitochondrial respiratory chain as a drug target

2.1. NADH-fumarate reductase system (fumarate respiration)

Since the 1970s, when albendazole became available for clinical use, no new drugs for echinococcosis have been identified, as mentioned above. As an efficient drug for AE is still not available, new chemotherapy targets are necessary [34, 35]. Our group has focused on the mitochondrial respiratory chain, namely the NADH-fumarate reductase system, of parasites as a potential drug target. Parasitic helminthes possess an NADH-fumarate reductase system that is highly adapted to anaerobic conditions [36, 37]. The parasitic nematode *Ascaris. suum* is a suitable model for biochemical studies of mitochondrial NADH-fumarate reductase systems because the body sizes of adult worms are easy to manipulate. We previously reported that the NADH-fumarate reductase system is a good target for the development of novel, selective anthelmintic compounds as modeled in *A. suum* [38, 39]. It is composed of complex I (NADH-quinone reductase, NQR), complex II (quinol-fumarate reductase, QFR), and a low-potential electron mediator, rhodoquinone (RQ). Low-potential RQ transfers the reducing equivalent of NADH via complex I to complex II, and succinate is ultimately produced by QFR activity of complex II. The merit of this system is ATP synthesis using the coupling site of complex I even in the absence of oxygen. QFR catalyzes the reduction of fumarate to succinate, while SQR (succinate-quinone reductase, used in mammalian systems) does the oxidation of succinate in the opposite direction (**Figure 1**). The NADH-fumarate reductase

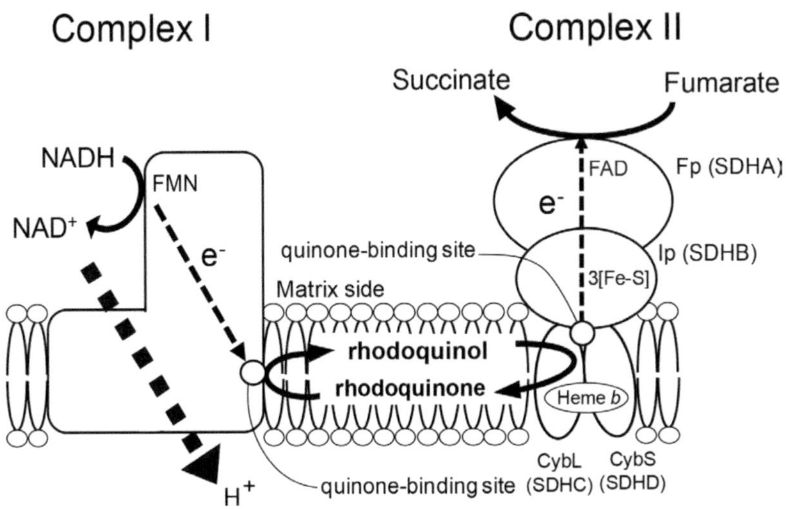

Figure 1. A schematic representation of the NADH-fumarate reductase system in adult *A. suum*, which catalyzes the last step of the phosphoenolpyruvate carboxykinase-succinate pathway. The NADH-fumarate reductase system is composed of complex I (NADH-quinone reductase), low-potential rhodoquinone (RQ), and complex II (quinol-fumarate reductase, QFR). In this system, electrons from NADH are transferred to RQ by the NADH-RQ reductase activity of mitochondrial complex I and then transferred to fumarate by the QFR activity of mitochondrial complex II through the quinone-binding site. Anaerobic electron transfer in complex I couples with proton transport across the mitochondrial inner membrane to generate ATP. *A. suum* complex II is composed of four subunits: flavoprotein subunit (Fp), iron-sulfur protein subunit (Ip), and cytochrome *b* large and small subunits (CybL and CybS, respectively). 3[Fe-S], iron-sulfur clusters; FAD, flavin adenine dinucleotide; and FMN, flavin mononucleotide.

system is absent in mammalian mitochondria living in aerobic conditions. Therefore, this unique respiratory system is considered to be a promising chemotherapeutic target for the development of novel anthelmintics.

2.2. Mitochondrial complex II

Complex II is a member of the tricarboxylic acid (TCA) cycle and respiratory chain. SQR as complex II catalyzes the oxidation of succinate to fumarate in the TCA cycle and transfers the electron to ubiquinone in the respiratory chain. QFR as complex II catalyzes the reduction of fumarate to succinate, a reverse reaction of succinate dehydrogenase (SDH), in the respiratory chain of mitochondria from anaerobic animals such as *A. suum* as described above. Generally, complex II consists of four subunits. Flavoprotein (Fp) subunit contains flavin adenine dinucleotide (FAD) as a prosthetic group and iron-sulfur protein (Ip) subunit contains three iron-sulfur (Fe-S) clusters [38]. The complex also contains large and small hydrophobic cytochrome *b* (CybL and CybS, respectively) subunits. The succinate-binding site is located in the Fp subunit, while the quinone-binding site is formed by the other three subunits, Ip, CybL, and CybS.

2.3. *E. multilocularis* complex II as a novel drug target

Our group has focused on the biochemical properties of complex II and its potential as a drug target against helminth infections [40–42]. This concept could be expanded to *Echinococcus* species, which belongs to parasitic platyhelminthes, distinct from nematodes. As expected, we found that the NADH-fumarate reductase system played a dominant role in isolated mitochondria from larval *E. multilocularis* [36]. In addition, quinazoline, an inhibitor of complex I, exhibited antiechinococcal activity under in vitro culture conditions [36]. These findings suggest that the NADH-fumarate reductase system is a potential therapeutic target in *E. multilocularis*. However, it is difficult to synthesize quinazoline derivatives. In addition, quinazoline and its derivatives exhibited strong toxicity in mammalian cells. Therefore, we focused on mitochondrial complex II in the NADH-fumarate reductase system as a drug target. Flutolanil and atpenin A5 are known effective inhibitors of the quinone-binding site of *A. suum* complex II [42, 43]. Elucidation of crystal structures of *A. suum* complex II in the presence of flutolanil provided useful information for the structure-based design of a more effective inhibitor [39, 44]. As a crystallographic analysis of *Echinococcus* complex II is challenging, we conducted comparative analyses of *E. multilocularis* with other parasites and host enzymes.

We cloned cDNA of complex II and assembly factors of *E. multilocularis* and purified subunits of complex II from mitochondria by high resolution clear native electrophoresis (hrCNE) to determine N-terminal amino acid sequences of mature subunits. In addition, we investigated the effects of several quinone-binding site inhibitors on *E. multilocularis* complex II.

3. Characterization of *E. multilocularis* complex II as a drug target

3.1. Cloning and sequence analyses of the genes for four constitutive subunits and two assembly factors

Since genome project data from Brehm and colleagues were released in advance on their website (Wellcome Trust Sanger Institute: http://www.sanger.ac.uk), we first identified complex II–related genes by BLAST search using human and other eukaryotic sequences as queries. A partial or full open reading frame (ORF) of four subunits composing mature complex II and two assembly factors were identified by TBLASTN search against expressed sequence tag (EST) or genomic contig and shotgun reads. Two isoforms were found for the Ip subunit, and the other subunits were encoded in a single gene each. Primers for the coding region of each gene were designed based on this information (**Table 1**). First, the coding region of the seven genes was amplified by gene-specific PCR, and sequences were determined after insertion into a cloning vector. For rapid amplification of cDNA ends (RACE) of 5′ and 3′ ends, new primers were designed from the confirmed coding regions. Finally, cDNA sequences of *sdha* (Fp), *sdhb1* (Ip1), *sdhb2* (Ip2), *sdhc* (CybL), *sdhd* (CybS), *sdhaf1*, and *sdhaf2* were determined (DDBJ accession numbers: AB699145–AB699151).

During 3′RACE of *sdhaf1*, we found that the first PCR yielded an exceptionally long amplified DNA fragment (ca. 1.4 kbp) compared to the ORF of *sdhaf1* (288 bp). Interestingly, this fragment contained another ORF homologous (27% of amino acid identity) to Tam41p in budding yeast (GenBank ID: NP_011560) [45], whose start codon overlapped the stop codon of *sdhaf1*. 3′RACE was conducted again with gene-specific primers complementary to the tam41 coding region, which is closer to the 3′-terminal end of cDNA compared to the initial 3′RACE

Primer		Sequences	Experiment
Fp-1	F	5′-AGGCTCCCAAGGCTGTTATC-3′	ORF
Fp-2	R	5′-GCAGACGTTCTGATCTAAAG-3′	ORF & 5′RACE 1st
Fp-3	F	5′-GCTTGCGCCCTCGATATT-3′	3′RACE 1st
Fp-4	F	5′-GTCTCATATGGAACTCGGAC-3′	3′RACE 2nd
Fp-5	R	5′-CGGAGTGAGCGACCGTATAGAG-3′	5′RACE 2nd
Fp-6	F	5′-CAGTTTTCGTGCACCTTCATGG-3′	ORF-full
Fp-7	R	5′-CCTTGAACGATTAGTAGGAACGG-3′	ORF-full
Ip1-1	F	5′-TCCGTTCTCTGCTTTTCGAC-3′	ORF & 3′RACE 1st
Ip1-2	R	5′-TCAGCATCTTCTTGATCTCACC-3′	ORF
Ip1-3	F	5′-TCTGCGCTATTCCCAAAGAT-3′	3′RACE 2nd
Ip1-4	R	5′-GGAATAGCGCAGAGACAGGCCAGAC-3′	5′RACE 1st
Ip1-5	R	5′-GAGCGTCAAGCATCATGGGAC-3′	5′RACE 2nd
Ip1-6	F	5′-TCGCCAGGAGAATGAATTCC-3′	ORF-full
Ip1-7	R	5′-GTCACTTCGAACCGGTTCAG-3′	ORF-full
Ip2-1	F	5′-GATAACTTGCAAGCGTGC-3′	3′RACE 1st
Ip2-2	F	5′-GTCCGGCTACATTGATACAC-3′	3′RACE 2nd
Ip2-3	R	5′-AATTTTGGTGACTTTATTGCTCCTC-3′	5′RACE 1st
Ip2-4	R	5′-AATGTGAGGGTTGGGTCGCAT-3′	5′RACE 2nd
Ip2-5	F	5′-GTGGTGGGAACATGAATTGTGTTTG-3′	ORF-full
Ip2-6	R	5′-GAATGCATCACAATGCCAGGA-3′	ORF-full
CybL-1	F	5′-TTTTTGCGAACGTTCTGTTG-3′	ORF & 3′RACE 1st
CybL-2	R	5′-CTTCCACAGGTCCGAACAC-3′	ORF
CybL-3	F	5′-AAGGGCAGCACAAGTGAGG-3′	3′RACE 2nd
CybL-4	R	5′-CCATGGCGACACCAGTAGCACGG-3′	5′RACE 1st
CybL-5	R	5′-AATATGTGAGGCGACCACGGG-3′	5′RACE 2nd
CybL-6	F	5′-GCGCGGTTAGACATGTCG-3′	ORF-full
CybL-7	R	5′-GGCTAGCAACATCTAGCTCCTG-3′	ORF-full
CybS-1	F	5′-ATGTCTTTCGCGCTTTTGG-3′	ORF
CybS-2	R	5′-TTTTGACGCCCTTAATAACACC-3′	ORF, 5′RACE 1st & 2nd
CybS-3	F	5′-GCGAAGTTGGGGACAGCT-3′	3′RACE 2nd
CybS-4	F	5′-GGCTTCATTGGCAGGATGTC-3′	ORF-full
CybS-5	R	5′-CACTGCGTGCTCAAAGAGACC-3′	ORF-full
AF1-1	F	5′-ATGTCTCGCCCATATAGTCAACTTC-3′	ORF & 3′RACE 1st
AF1-2	R	5′-TTAATCTTGTTTATGGGGAGGAAAAG-3′	ORF & 5′RACE 1st
AF1-3	F	5′-GACAGGTTCTGAAGCTCTATAAGGA-3′	3′RACE 2nd

Primer		Sequences	Experiment
AF1-4	F	5′-ATATGGGGTCGTTGGTTATG-3′	3′RACE 1st
AF1-5	F	5′-AGTAGAGACGCCAATCACCACGA-3′	3′RACE2nd
AF1-6	R	5′-GACCTGCCTCAAGGTCTTCC-3′	5′RACE 2nd
AF1-7	F	5′-TTGATTATTAGCGCAATATAAGGTG-3′	ORF-full
AF1-8	R	5′-TTTTCTAAATGTTTTATTCAGGCAAA-3′	ORF-full
AF2-1	F	5′-ATGGTGCTGTCTCTTAATCGTTTGAC-3′	ORF & 3′RACE 1st
AF2-2	R	5′-CTACACAGTGTGGGGGTGAATATTG-3′	ORF & 5′RACE 1st
AF2-3	F	5′-TCTGTTGCGACAATGAGGAG-3′	3′RACE 2nd
AF2-4	R	5′-TCTGTTGCGACAATGAGGAG-3′	5′RACE 2nd
AF2-5	F	5′-ACTATTAAACTTTCTGCTTGGTTGCAT-3′	ORF-full
AF2-6	R	5′-GTTGTATATAATGCTGTAATTAACTAATAGGACAAC-3′	ORF-full

Table 1. Gene-specific primers used in this chapter.

experiment. The presence of this polycistronic mRNA was confirmed by PCR with primers that were complementary to the 5′ untranslated region (UTR) of *sdhaf1* and 3′ UTR of tam41.

The number of amino acids of all determined proteins and their sequence identities with corresponding proteins in *A. suum* and humans are summarized in **Table 2**. The position from the first methionine (Met) of the N-terminal sequences of the four subunits in mature complex II is also listed in parentheses next to these 10 amino acids' sequences in **Table 3**. The two isoforms of Ip share the same sequence in this region. Two isoforms of Ip were reported in the parasitic nematode *Haemonchus contortus* [46]. Additionally, there are two isoforms of Fp, type I and II, in human complex II. It is speculated that complex II with type II Fp has a higher QFR activity and plays an important role in fumarate respiration in human mitochondria as the terminal oxidase of the system [38]. Isoforms of *E. multilocularis* Ip might be related to

			Identity of amino acid sequence (%)	
Gene	**Product**	**Amino acids**	**A. suum (adult)**	**Human**
sdha	Fp	647	68	72
sdhb1	Ip1	282	58	62
sdhb2	Ip2	282	57	62
sdhc	CybL	194	23	31
sdhd	CybS	153	27	30
sdhaf1	SDHAF1	95	27	39
sdhaf2	SDHAF2	140	31	41

Table 2. Summary of cloning and translated amino acid sequence.

Gene	Product	Amino acid of premature protein (upper) N-terminal amino acid of mature protein (positions*)
sdha	Fp	MAFLVRASFASFAARLGCLPTFAGASRHVSTVGKDYTI
		VSTVGKDYTI (29–38)
sdhb1	Ip1	MNSVLCFSTRYACVIGQTARYASTGPVMKKF
		ASTGPVMKKF (22–31)
sdhb2	Ip2	MNCVCSLSLRFEFLLIQTARYASTGPVMKKF
		ASTGPVMKKF (22–31)
sdhc	CybL	MSVFANVLLRAHAAPFRGVAARNLSMALQPLLLRTAPVLSATKHYKGSTSEEVRL
		KGSTSEEVRL (46–55)
sdhd	CybS	MSFALLASKHLIRRAAVSSFVSANACRTLVCTPNNKAKLGTAPQPV
		AKLGTAPQPV (37–46)

*Positions of the N-terminal 10 amino acids from the first Met in cDNA.

Table 3. N-terminal amino acid.

changes in the respiration system, although the expression ratio of the two isoforms must be estimated during the life cycle.

3.2. Purification of *E. multilocularis* complex II by electrophoresis

As all the genes for mitochondrial complex II are chromosomally encoded and the N-terminal of each peptide is processed during mitochondrial localization, *E. multilocularis* complex II was partially purified and N-terminal amino acid sequences of the subunits were determined. Mitochondrial samples solubilized and separated by hrCNE were further subjected to two-dimensional SDS-PAGE (see Section 5). Since first-dimensional electrophoresis was conducted by hrCNE, the four subunits of complex II were expected to align under the SDH activity stained band (**Figure 2A**). Based on the apparent molecular weight, candidates of the four subunits were selected (indicated by black arrows): Fp (75 kDa), Ip (28 kDa), CybL (15 kDa), and CybS (12 kDa) (**Figure 2B**). Bands corresponding to these subunits in protoscoleces (larval stage) and adult *E. multilocularis* were detected at the same positions. From the partially purified sample, four subunits could be stained by coomassie brilliant blue (CBB), and N-terminal amino acid sequences were determined in 10 residues for those four bands (**Table 3**).

3.3. Inhibition of complex II by flutolanil, atpenin A5, and ascofuranone

We developed a method to separate *E. multilocularis* mitochondria to study its biochemical properties, including inhibitor screening. We constructed a quinone-binding site inhibitor library since this site is considered a good target for antiparasitic drugs. The inhibitory effect of flutolanil, atpenin A5, and ascofuranone as representative inhibitors was subsequently analyzed.

http://dx.doi.org/10.5772/intechopen.68565

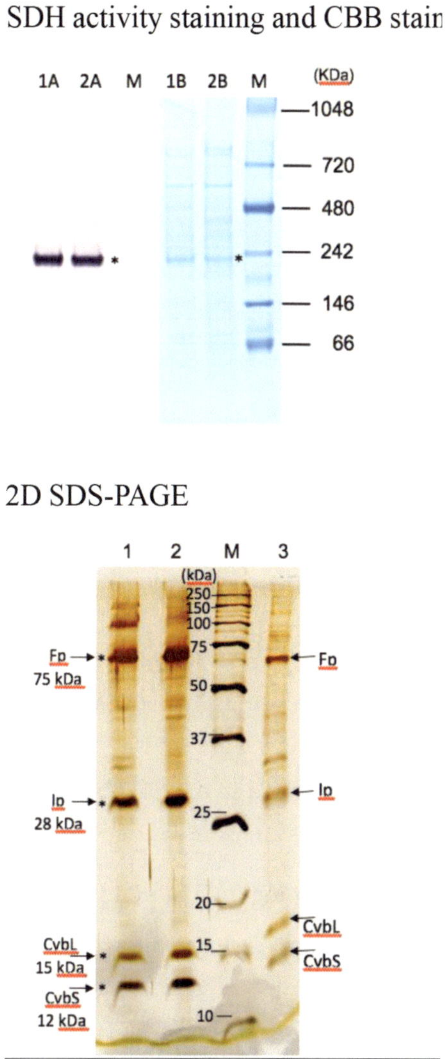

Figure 2. A SDH (succinate dehydrogenase) activity staining. Lane 1A: adult *E. multilocularis* and lane 2A: protoscoleces (PSC). CBB (Coomassie Brilliant Blue) staining. Lane 1B: adult *E. multilocularis* and lane 2B: PSC. Asterisks indicate complex II. Lane M: molecular weight markers. B. 2D SDS-PAGE. Comparison of (1) PSC complex II, (2) adult complex II, (3) purified *A. suum* complex II, and (M) molecular weight markers. Candidates of four subunits were selected (indicated by black arrows), which correspond to flavoprotein (Fp, 75 kDa), iron-sulfur cluster protein (Ip, 28 kDa), cytochrome *b* large subunit (CybL, 15 kDa), and cytochrome *b* small subunits (CybS, 12 kDa). Asterisks indicate PSC complex II subunits. PSC and adult complex II subunits demonstrated similar sizes.

The 50% inhibitory concentration (IC_{50}) values of flutolanil, atpenin A5, and ascofuranone for *E. multilocularis* QFR are shown in **Table 4**. The selectivity index was expressed with the IC_{50} of each inhibitor for porcine SQR. The IC_{50} and selectivity index of flutolanil for *E. multilocularis* QFR were 15 μM and 2.9, respectively (IC_{50} of porcine SQR was 44 μM), while the IC_{50} and selectivity index of flutolanil for *A. suum* QFR were 0.058 μM and 758, respectively [44]. The IC_{50} of atpenin A5 for porcine SQR (0.0036 μM) was lower than that for *E. multilocularis* (0.059 μM) and *A. suum* QFR (0.012 μM) [43]. Surprisingly, the IC_{50} and selectivity index of ascofuranone,

Inhibitor	IC_{50} (μM)			Selectivity index
	E. multilocularis QFR	*A. suum* QFR	Porcine SQR	Porcin IC_{50}/*E. multilocularis* IC_{50}
Flutolanil	15 ± 0.28	0.058*	44	2.9
Atpenin A5	0.059 ± 0.0063	0.012**	0.0036	0.061
Ascofuranone	0.85 ± 0.070	10	300	350

*Harada et al. Biochimica et Biophysica Acta. 2013;1827:658-667.
**Miyadera et al. Proceedings of the National Academy of the Sciences USA. 2003;21:473-477.

Table 4. The inhibitory effect of representative quinone-binding site inhibitors.

which was developed as an antitrypanosomal drug, for *E. multilocularis* QFR, were 0.85 μM and 350, respectively, although the IC_{50} of ascofuranone for *A. suum* QFR was 10 μM.

4. Discussion

4.1. Features of *E. multilocularis* complex II

In this chapter, the molecular characterization of *E. multilocularis* complex II was performed, including complex II inhibitor screening.

The FAD prosthetic group of Fp is localized in the FAD-binding domain by a covalent bond to histidine (His) and hydrogen bonds with highly conserved residues across amino acid sequences of complex II from various species [44, 47]. Fp in *E. multilocularis* has this conserved sequence, including the segment containing FAD-bound His.

The Ip subunit generally contains three Fe-S clusters coordinated by cysteine (Cys) residues [10]. The Ip subunit of *E. multilocularis* also has three well-conserved Cys-rich regions associated with the Fe-S cluster. An unusual amino acid substitution was found in the Fe-S cluster related to the Cys-rich region. A comparison of this amino acid with the known crystal structure of complex II placed it spatially in the vicinity of the 4Fe-4S center. We found two isoforms of *E. multilocularis* Ip (EmIp1 and EmIp2), which differ from each other by remarkable one amino acid residue. Leucine (Leu) 180 of EmIp1 and phenylalanine (Phe) 180 of EmIp2 are very rare substitutions in the second conserved Cys-rich region among complex II. This position is primarily an alanine (Ala), and infrequently a glycine, in bacterial or eukaryotic enzymes. Ala is generally located adjacent to the second conserved Cys in the second Cys-rich region of Ip, interacting with the Fe-S cluster in many species. *E. multilocularis* complex II functions as QFR with RQ as the electron donor. Interestingly, *Rhodospirillum rubrum*, a photosynthetic bacterium that we consider as a candidate expression host for *E. multilocularis* complex II, has a Phe at this position, similar to EmIp2. Because *R. rubrum* has RQ and ubiquinone as hydrophobic electron carriers in the cytoplasmic membrane, its complex II may function as QFR, utilizing RQ similar to *E. multilocularis*. Cloning of *sdhb* (Ip) highlighted the features of *E. multilocularis* complex II. The role of this amino acid residue in the catalytic activity will be studied in future mutational analyses of *E. multilocularis* and *R. rubrum* complex II.

In our chapter, mitochondrial complex II of *E. multilocularis* was purified by preparative hrCNE, and N-terminal amino acid sequences of all four subunits from mature enzymes were determined. The benefit of employing preparative hrCNE is that the loss of protein during the experiment is small since the condition is already fixed by analysis on a minigel. Purification starting with 2.6 mg of mitochondrial protein successfully yielded a sufficient amount of purified complex II for subsequent protein sequencing analysis.

4.2. Identification of *sdhaf1* and *sdhaf2*

Functional expression of eukaryotic complex II in other organisms is difficult because complex II is a multi-subunit enzyme, and many prosthetic groups, such as FAD, are associated with this enzyme. In this condition, two important proteins, succinate dehydrogenase assembly factor 1 (*SDHAF1*) and *SDHAF2* (*SDHAF2*, or *SDH5*), involved in the synthesis of functional complex II were reported. Their gene products are not the components of mature complex II [48–50]. SDHAF1 is suggested to play an essential role in complex II assembly. SDHAF2 may be required for the insertion of FAD cofactor into Fp. Coexpression of these genes with the four subunits present in mature complex II may be required for functional expression of eukaryotic complex II in heterologous expression systems such as bacteria.

Although *sdhaf2* of *A. suum* and *Caenorhabditis elegans* was annotated, *sdhaf1* has not been annotated in the EST database [https://www.ncbi.nlm.nih.gov/nucest] or WormBase [http://www.wormbase.org]. Furthermore, the genome annotation of *sdhaf1* has not been assigned in the draft genome sequence and transcriptome analysis of *Echinococcus* [51]. TBLASTN search using human and other eukaryotic sequences as queries in WormBase [http://www.wormbase.org/tools/blast_blat] against the genome detected the *sdhaf1* candidate region as an intron-less structure on chromosome V, corresponding to positions 4710485–4710739 (genomic position: 4710485–4710739). In the EST database, the corresponding sequence was found as an ORF before the start codon of *cif-1*, an ortholog of human eukaryotic translation initiation factor 3, and ORF in several mRNA variants of *cif-1* (e.g., yk1259f02.5). However, *cif-1* itself is not related to complex II or Tam41P. BLASTP search in WormBase did not yield the sequence found in the genome and EST. Taken together, *sdhaf1* found in *C. elegans* genome and its expression was observed, although not annotated. A homologous gene was also found in *A. suum* (GenBank ID: JI213553). After the first report of SDHAF1 and SDHAF2, several studies have reported SDHAF2 but not SDHAF1. Identification of the prokaryotic gene corresponding to *sdhaf2*, named *sdhE* in prokaryotes, suggests a common role of this gene for the assembly process of the complex II. However, *sdhaf1* was not annotated as a protein coding gene in WormBase, which is one of the best organized and updated genes and protein databases for *C. elegans*. Cloning of *E. multilocularis sdhaf1* revealed polycistronic expression of this gene with downstream tam41. The same genome structure was conserved in *Schistosoma mansoni*, the first genomic reference for Platyhelminthes. A homologous ORF was identified in *C. elegans* EST database as a part of *cif-1* mRNA. Considering the small size of this gene (<300 bp) and the gene arrangement in *E. multilocularis* and *S. mansoni*, transcription in a polycistronic manner in *C. elegans* does not necessary indicate a correlation between *sdhaf1* and *cif-1*. However, because of its small size and mRNA structure, this gene might have been overlooked in this organism.

4.3. Inhibition of complex II by a quinone-binding site inhibitor

An inhibitor of the mitochondrial respiratory chain, atovaquone, has been used as an antimalarial agent [52]. Thus, it is reasonable to identify potent and specific inhibitors for the respiratory chain of *E. multilocularis*. Flutolanil, a commercially available fungicide, specifically inhibits helminth complex II [42]. The IC_{50} and selectivity index of flutolanil for *A. suum* were 58 nM and 762, respectively. The flutolanil-binding site is located at the RQ-binding pocket, which is formed at the interface domain composed of three subunits, Ip, CybL, and CybS [39, 44]. Moreover, CH-π interaction between flutolanil isopropyl group and tryptophan69 (Trp) in CybL is one of the significant factors for the highly specific inhibitory effects of flutolanil against *A. suum* complex II [44]. Our finding that Trp69 is replaced with methionine (Met) in *E. multilocularis* and human (arrow A in **Figure 3**) likely explains why complex II activity in *E. multilocularis* was not inhibited by flutolanil. In fact, Harada et al. reported that porcine complex II is resistant to flutolanil since Trp69 is replaced by Met in porcine CybL [44]. Furthermore, in *E. multilocularis*, a phenylalanine (Phe) is located four amino acids downstream of the Met (arrow B in **Figure 3**). This Phe is replaced with isoleucine in human. This information is useful for the design of selective inhibitors of *E. multilocularis* complex II because the Phe residue forms a strong interaction, such as CH-π or cation-π interaction, with the inhibitor [53, 54].

```
                                     (A) (B)
                                      ↓   ↓
E.m CybL    NIKLKRPWSPHILIYSPPLCMRNSFLHRATG   98
Hum CybL    NIGSNRPLSPHITIYSWSLPMAMSICHRGTG   75
A.s CybL    QRALKRPIAPHLTIYKPQMTWMVSGLHRVTG   79
```

Figure 3. A comparison of the amino acid sequence of cytochrome *b* large subunit (CybL) from *E. multilocularis* (*E. m*), human (Hum), and *A. suum* (*A. s*). The arrow A indicates that tryptophan at position 69 is replaced with methionine in *E. multilocularis* and human. The arrow B indicates the phenylalanine four amino acids downstream of the methionine at arrow A in *E. multilocularis* is changed to isoleucine in human.

Interestingly, ascofuranone, which is a specific quinone-binding site inhibitor of cyanide-insensitive trypanosome alternative oxidase in *Trypanosoma brucei* mitochondria [55, 56], inhibited *E. multilocularis* QRF at the nanomolar order. To our knowledge, this study is the first to demonstrate that ascofuranone acts as a complex II inhibitor. Furthermore, our preliminary study showed ascofuranone has the ability to kill protoscoleces in culture within several days (data not shown). Our findings may aid in the development of new targeted therapy against *Echinococcus* complex II. We have synthesized more than 400 ascofuranone derivatives and will evaluate the structure-activity relationship in in vitro and in vivo studies.

5. Experimental information

5.1. Isolation of *E. multilocularis* protoscoleces and preparation of enriched mitochondrial fractions

The Nemuro strain of *E. multilocularis*, which is maintained at biosafety level 3 in the Hokkaido Institute of Public Health (Sapporo, Japan), was used in this study. The mitochondria of protoscoleces were prepared as described previously [36]. To isolate protoscoleces, the mature larval parasites were minced with scissors, pushed through a metal mesh, and washed repeatedly with physiological saline. The isolated protoscolex sediment was suspended in 5 volumes of mitochondrial preparation buffer (210 mM mannitol, 10 mM sucrose, 1 mM disodium EDTA, and 50 mM Tris-HCl [pH 7.5]), supplemented with 10 mM sodium malonate. The parasite materials were homogenized with a motor-driven glass/glass homogenizer. The homogenate was diluted with the mitochondrial preparation buffer to 10 times the volume of the original protoscolex sediment and then centrifuged at 800 × *g* for 10 min to precipitate cell debris and nuclei. The supernatant was then centrifuged at 8000 × *g* for 10 min to obtain the mitochondrial pellet. The pellet was resuspended in mitochondrial preparation buffer (without malonate) and centrifuged at 12,000 × *g* for 10 min. The enriched mitochondrial fraction was suspended in mitochondrial preparation buffer (without malonate) [36].

5.2. hrCNE and two-dimensional SDS-PAGE

Separation profile of complex II by hrCNE was analyzed and the condition for purification was optimized by isocratic acrylamide minigel. The mitochondrial membrane of *E. multilocularis* was suspended as 10 mg/mL protein in gel buffer (50 mM Tris-HCl, pH 8.0). The membrane was solubilized by the addition of 50 mM Tris-HCl (pH 8.0), 4% SML (sucrose monolaurate), 40% (v/v) glycerol, and 2 mM sodium malonate on ice followed by centrifugation (200,000 × *g*, 4°C, 30 min). The supernatant was mixed with 1/10 volume of loading dye (50% glycerol and 0.1% Ponceau S), and 55 μL of the resulting solution was applied to the well. Anode buffer (20 × running buffer) and cathode buffer (20 × running buffer, 0.02% n-dodecyl-β-D-maltoside, and 0.05% sodium deoxycholate) were used irrespective of the detergent for solubilization. Electrophoresis was performed in a cold room (4°C), starting with 100 and 250 V constant voltage for 1 h. The complex II band was visualized by GelCode Blue Safe Protein Stain (Thermo Scientific) or SDH activity staining. For activity staining, a gel strip was soaked in 10 mL of 5 mM Tris-HCl (pH 7.4) containing 25 mg of nitro blue tetrazolium, and then the reaction was started by the addition of 150 μL of 4 mg/mL phenazine methosulfate and 200 μL of 1 M sodium succinate. The complex II band was detected by activity staining and cut from the one-dimensional gel (CBB staining). The gel was equilibrated with SDS-PAGE buffer and then loaded onto the two-dimensional gel (4.5% acrylamide, 0.12% bisacrylamide, 0.25 M Tris-HCl (pH 6.8), 0.4% sodium dodecyl sulfate, 0.05% ammonium persulfate, and *N,N,N',N'*-tetramethylethylenediamine). Protein spots were visualized by silver staining (2D-Silver Stain-II kit, Cosmo Bio).

5.3. Partial purification of complex II by preparative hrCNE

Prepforesis® (ATTO) was used for preparative hrCNE. Separation gel (8% acrylamide) was prepared in a 1.6-cm diameter column at 2-cm height, and sample gel (3% acrylamide) was layered at 1-cm height. For solubilization, 2.6-mg protein of *E. multilocularis* mitochondria was precipitated, resuspended in 300 μL of solubilization buffer (10 mM Tris-HCl, 0.5 M 6-aminohexanoic acid, 5% (v/v) glycerol, 2.5% digitonin, pH 8.0), and kept on ice for 1 h. The resulting suspension was centrifuged (200,000 × *g*, 10 min), and 3 μL of loading dye was added to the supernatant. The buffer system was the same as that of the minigel and kept at 6°C by a circulator. Electrophoresis was performed at 10 mA. The volume of one fraction was approximately 650 μL and 50 fractions were collected.

5.4. N-terminal amino acid determination of complex II constitutive subunits

Complex II-containing fractions from hrCNE were individually concentrated to approximately 70 μL by Amicon Ultra-4 Centrifugal Filter Units (molecular weight cutoff is 50,000). After rough estimation of the concentration and purity of complex II on SDS-PAGE with silver staining, protein was precipitated with trichloroacetic acid. Briefly, 30 μL of water and 10 μL of 100% (w/v) trichloroacetic acid solution were added to 60 μL of concentrated fraction and then the mixture was incubated on ice for 15 min and sedimented (14,000 × *g* for 10 min). These samples were then subjected to 12.5% SDS-PAGE, and proteins were transferred to an Immobilon-P membrane (Millipore), followed by staining with CBB G-250. Ten amino acid residues were determined with a Procise 494 cLC Protein Sequencing System (Applied Biosystems) at APRO Life Science Institute (Tokushima, Japan).

5.5. cDNA synthesis and cloning of complex II–related genes

Frozen mature larval parasites were pulverized with a mortar and pestle in liquid nitrogen, and total RNA was prepared using TRIzol LS Reagent (Invitrogen), according to the manufacturer's protocols, followed by further purification with RNeasy (Qiagen) and DNase I treatment. For 5′RACE, cDNA was synthesized with the SMART™ RACE cDNA Amplification Kit (Clontech) using ReverTra Ace (Toyobo) as a reverse transcriptase. For 3′RACE, the oligo(dT) primer 5′-GACTCGAGTCGACATCGA$(T)_{17}$-3′ was used for cDNA synthesis.

Primer sets to amplify the partial coding region of each subunit (except *sdhb2*) were designed based on the TBLASTN search, which was performed against the database of *E. multilocularis* EST or genomic contig and shotgun reads [http://www.sanger.ac.uk/cgi-bin/blast/submitblast/Echinococcus]. PCR was performed using Takara Ex Taq (Takara Bio) or PfuUltra II Fusion HS DNA polymerase (Stratagene). Gene-specific primers for 5′RACE and 3′RACE were designed from determined sequences in the coding region. For *sdhb2*, gene-specific primers were designed from the genomic contig (**Table 1**). All RACE experiments were performed as first PCR and nested PCR to obtain sufficient amplification of the DNA fragments. The universal primers for the first PCR and nested PCR for 5′RACE were universal primer mix and nested universal primers, respectively, which were provided within the SMART™ RACE cDNA Amplification Kit. For 3′RACE, the adaptor primer 5′-GACTCGAGTCGACATCG-3′ was used for both first and nested PCRs as the universal primer. These products were separated by electrophoresis on agarose gel, and target products were extracted with the MagExtractor-PCR & Gel Clean up kit (Toyobo). The gel-purified products were inserted into the pGEM-T vector (Promega) after A-tailing with Taq polymerase (Invitrogen) for sequencing. Entire ORFs were amplified using primers complementary to the determined 5′ UTR and 3′ UTR, and sequences were confirmed.

5.6. Enzyme inhibition assays

QFR and SQR assays were performed as described previously [36]. The final mitochondrial protein concentration was 50 μg/mL of the reaction mixture. QFR and SQR activities were assayed under anaerobic and aerobic conditions, respectively. QFR and SQR activities were determined by monitoring the absorbance change of decyl RQ (60 μM) at 340 nm and ubiquinone-2 (60 μM) at 278 nm (using SHIMADZU spectrophotometer UV-3000), respectively. We determined IC_{50} values of the quinone-binding site inhibitors against QFR activity of the mitochondria of protoscoleces. Flutolanil (Wako), atpenin A5 (ENZO Life Sciences), and ascofuranone were used in the assays (**Figure 4**). Ascofuranone was obtained from Align Pharmaceutical.

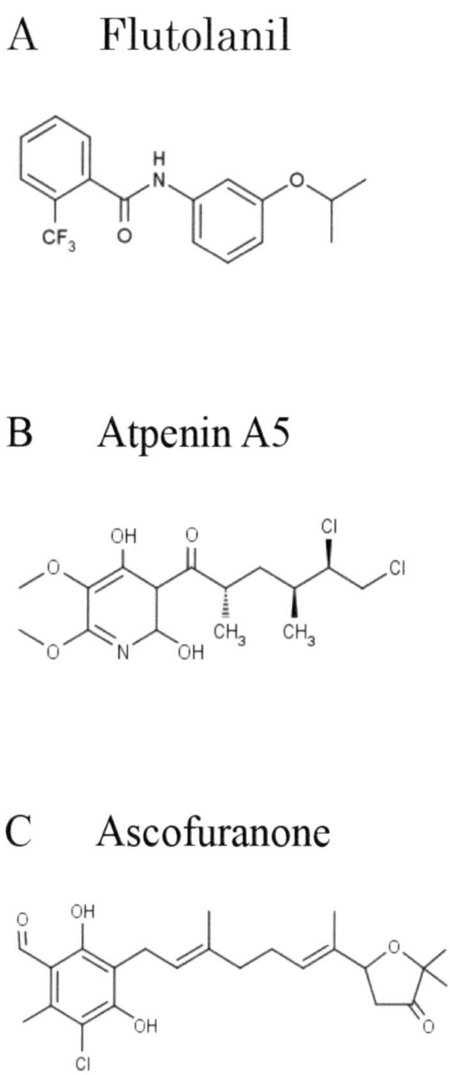

Figure 4. The chemical structure of inhibitors of the quinone-binding site. A. Flutolanil, a competitive inhibitor of the quinone-binding site of *A. suum* complex II. B. Atpenin A5, a competitive inhibitor of the quinone-binding site of complex II of many species. C. Ascofuranone, a potent inhibitor of cyanide-insensitive alternative oxidase of *Trypanosoma brucei*.

Acknowledgements

This work was supported in part by a grant-in-aid for Infectious Disease Control from the Science and Technology Research Partnership for Sustainable Development (no. 10000284 to KK), a grant-in-aid for the Bilateral Joint Research Project from the Japan Society for the Promotion of Science (no. 16035611-000722 to KK), and a grant from the Program for the Promotion of Basic and Applied Research for Innovations in Bio-Oriented Industries (to KK).

Author details

Shigehiro Enkai[1,2]*, Kimitoshi Sakamoto[1,3], Miho Kaneko[1,4], Hirokazu Kouguchi[5], Takao Irie[5], Kinpei Yagi[5], Yuka Ishida[6], Jun Matsumoto[7], Yuzaburo Oku[8], Ken Katakura[9], Osamu Fujita[10], Tomoyoshi Nozaki[11,12] and Kiyoshi Kita[1,2]

*Address all correspondence to: enkai@nagasaki-u.ac.jp

1 Department of Biomedical Chemistry, Graduate School of Medicine, The University of Tokyo, Tokyo, Japan

2 Nagasaki University School of Tropical Medicine and Global Health, Nagasaki, Japan

3 Department of Biochemistry and Molecular Biology, Faculty of Agriculture and Life Science, Hirosaki University, Hirosaki, Japan

4 Department of Hygiene and Molecular Epidemiology, Graduate School of Biomedical Sciences, Nagasaki University, Nagasaki, Japan

5 Department of Infectious Diseases, Hokkaido Institute of Public Health, Sapporo, Hokkaido, Japan

6 Atto Corporation, Tokyo, Japan

7 Laboratory of Medical Zoology, Department of Veterinary Medicine, College of Bioresource Sciences, Nihon University, Fujisawa, Japan

8 Laboratory of Parasitology, School of Veterinary Medicine, Faculty of Agriculture, Tottori University, Tottori, Japan

9 Laboratory of Parasitology, Department of Disease Control, Graduate School of Veterinary Medicine, Hokkaido University, Sapporo, Japan

10 Department of Veterinary Science, National Institute of Infectious Diseases, Toyama, Tokyo, Japan

11 Department of Parasitology, National Institute of Infectious Diseases, Toyama, Tokyo, Japan

12 Graduate School of Life and Environmental Sciences, University of Tsukuba, Tsukuba, Ibaraki, Japan

References

[1] Rinaldi F, Brunetti E, Neumayr A, Maestri M, Goblirsch S, Tamarozzi F. Cystic echinococcosis of the liver: A primer for hepatologists. World Journal of Hepatology. 2014;**6**: 293-305. DOI: 10.4254/wjh.v6.i5.293

[2] WHO Informal Working Group. International classification of ultrasound images in cystic echinococcosis for application in clinical and field epidemiological settings. Acta Tropica. 2003;**85**:253-261. DOI: 10.1016/S0001706X(02)002231

[3] Mihmanli M, Idiz UO, Kaya C, Demir U, Bostanci O, Omeroglu S, Bozkurt E. Current status of diagnosis and treatment of hepatic echinococcosis. World Journal of Hepatology. 2016;**8**:1169-1181. DOI: 10.4254/wjh.v8.i28.1169

[4] Filice C, Brunetti E. Use of PAIR in human cystic echinococcosis. Acta Tropica. 1997;**64**: 95-107. DOI: 10.1016/S0001706X(96)006420

[5] Buttenschoen K, Carli Buttenschoen D, Gruener B, Kern P, Beger HG, HenneBruns D, Reuter S. Longterm experience on surgical treatment of alveolar echinococcosis. Langenbecks Archive of Surgery. 2009;**394**:689-698. DOI: 10.1007/s00423-008-0392-5

[6] Brunetti E, Kern P, Vuitton DA. Expert consensus for the diagnosis and treatment of cystic and alveolar echinococcosis in humans. Acta Tropica. 2010;**114**:1-16. DOI: 10.1016/j.actatropica.2009.11.001

[7] Reuter S, Jensen B, Buttenschoen K, Kratzer W, Kern P. Benzimi dazoles in the treatment of alveolar echinococcosis: A comparative study and review of the literature. Journal of Antimicrobial Chemotherapy. 2000;**46**:451-456. DOI: 10.1093/jac/46.3.451

[8] Ammann RW, Hirsbrunner R, Cotting J, Steiger U, Jacquier P, Eckert J. Recurrence rate after discontinuation of longterm mebendazole therapy in alveolar echinococcosis (preliminary results). The American Journal of Tropical Medicine and Hygiene. 1990;**43**:506-515

[9] Ammann RW, Ilitsch N, Marincek B, Freiburghaus AU. Effect of chemotherapy on the larval mass and the longterm course of alveolar echinococcosis. Swiss Echinococcosis Study Group. Hepatology. 1994;**19**:735-742. DOI: 10.1002/hep.1840190328

[10] Horton RJ. Albendazole in treatment of human cystic echinococcosis:12 years of experience. Acta Tropica. 1997;**64**:79-93. DOI: 10.1016/S0001-706X(96)00640-7

[11] Taylor DH, Morris DL, Richards KS, Reffin D. *Echinococcus multilocularis*: In vivo results of therapy with albendazole and praziquantel. Transactions of the Royal Society of Tropical Medicine and Hygiene. 1988;**82**:611-615

[12] Yuan M, Luo Y, Xin Q, Gao H, Zhang G, Jing T. Efficacy of osthole for *Echinococcus granulosus* in vitro and *Echinococcus multilocularis* in vivo. Veterinary Parasitology. 2016;**226**:38-43. DOI: 10.1016/j.vetpar.2016.05.016

[13] Albani CM, Pensel PE, Elissondo N, Gambino G, Elissondo MC. In vivo activity of albendazole in combination with thymol against *Echinococcus multilocularis*. Veterinary Parasitology. 2015;**212**:193-199. DOI: 10.1016/j.vetpar.2015.06.030

[14] Stadelmann B, Rufener R, Aeschbacher D, Spiliotis M, Gottstein B, Hemphill A. Screening of the Open Source Malaria Box Reveals an Early Lead Compound for the Treatment of Alveolar Echinococcosis. PLoS Neglected Tropical Diseases. 2016;**10**:e0004535. DOI: 10.1371/journal.pntd.0004535

[15] Kern P, Abboud P, Kern W, Stich A, BressonHadni S, Guerin B, Buttenschoen K, Gruener B, Reuter S, Hemphill A. Critical appraisal of nitazoxanide for the treatment of alveolar echinococcosis. American Journal of Tropical Medicine and Hygiene. 2008;**79**:119

[16] Woollard DJ, Gauci CG, Heath DD, Lightowlers MW. Epitope specificities and antibody responses to the EG95 hydatid vaccine. Parasite Immunology. 1998;**20**:535-540 DOI: 10.1046/j.1365-3024.1998.00176.x

[17] Chow C, Gauci CG, Cowman AF, Lightowlers MW. A gene family expressing a host-protective antigen of *Echinococcus granulosus*. Molecular and Biochemical Parasitology. 2001;**118**:83-88. DOI: 10.1016/S0166-6851(01)00373-5

[18] Larrieu E, Mujica G, Gauci CG, Vizcaychipi K, Seleiman M, Herrero E, Labanchi JL, Araya D, Sepúlveda L, Grizmado C, Calabro A, Talmon G, Poggio TV, Crowley P, Cespedes G, Santillán G, García Cachau M, Lamberti R, Gino L, Donadeu M, Lightowlers MW. Pilot Field Trial of the EG95 Vaccine Against Ovine Cystic Echinococcosis in Rio Negro, Argentina: Second Study of Impact. PLoS Neglected Tropical Diseases. 2015;**9**:e0004134. DOI: 10.1371/journal.pntd.0004134

[19] Gauci C, Merli M, Muller V, Chow C, Yagi K, Mackenstedt U, Lightowlers MW. Molecular cloning of a vaccine antigen against infection with the larval stage of *Echinococcus multilocularis*. Infection and Immunity. 2002;**70**:3969-3972 DOI: 10.1128/IAI.70.7.3969-3972.2002

[20] Kouguchi H, Matsumoto J, Katoh Y, Oku Y, Suzuki T, Yagi K: The vaccination potential of EMY162 antigen against *Echinococcus multilocularis* infection. Biochemical Biophysical Research Communications. 2007;**363**:915-920. DOI: 10.1016/j.bbrc.2007.09.023

[21] Katoh Y, Kouguchi H, Matsumoto J, Goto A, Suzuki T, Oku Y, Yagi K. Characterization of emY162 encoding an immunogenic protein cloned from an adult worm-specific cDNA library of *Echinococcus multilocularis*. Biochimica et Biophysica Acta. 2008;**1780**:1-6. DOI: 10.1016/j.bbagen.2007.08.020

[22] Li Y, Liu X, Zhu Y, Zhou X, Cao C, Hu X, Ma H, Wen H, Ma X, Ding JB. Bioinformatic prediction of epitopes in the Emy162 antigen of *Echinococcus multilocularis*. Experimental and Therapeutic Medicine. 2013;**6**:335-340. DOI: 10.3892/etm.2013.1142

[23] Zhang F, Ma X, Zhu Y, Wang H, Liu X, Zhu M, Ma H, Wen H, Fan H, Ding J. Identification, expression and phylogenetic analysis of EgG1Y162 from *Echinococcus granulosus*. International Journal of Clinical and Experimental Pathology. 2014;**7**:5655-5664

[24] Dang Z, Yagi K, Oku Y, Kouguchi H, Kajino K, Watanabe J, Matsumoto J, Nakao R, Wakaguri H, Toyoda A, Sugimoto C. Evaluation of *Echinococcus multilocularis* tetraspanins as vaccine candidates against primary alveolar echinococcosis. Vaccine. 2009;**27**:7339-7345. DOI: 10.1016/j.vaccine.2009.09.045

[25] Dang Z, Yagi K, Oku Y, Kouguchi H, Kajino K, Matsumoto J, Nakao R, Wakaguri H, Toyoda A, Yin H, Sugimoto C. A pilot study on developing mucosal vaccine against alveolar echinococcosis (AE) using recombinant tetraspanin 3: Vaccine efficacy and immunology. PLoS Neglected Tropical Diseases. 2012;**6**:e1570. DOI: 10.1371/journal.pntd.0001570

[26] Hu D, Song X, Xie Y, Zhong X, Wang N, Zheng Y, Gu X, Wang T, Peng X, Yang G. Molecular insights into a tetraspanin in the hydatid tapeworm *Echinococcus granulosus*. Parasites & Vectors. 2015;**8**:311. DOI: 10.1186/s13071-015-0926-y

[27] Petavy AF, Hormaeche C, Lahmar S, Ouhelli H, Chabalgoity A, Marchal T, Azzouz S, Schreiber F, Alvite G, Sarciron ME, Maskell D, Esteves A, Bosquet G. An oral recombinant vaccine in dogs against *Echinococcus granulosus*, the causative agent of human hydatid disease: A pilot study. PLoS Neglected Tropical Diseases. 2008;**2**:e125. DOI: 10.1371/journal.pntd.0000125

[28] Zhang W, Zhang Z, Shi B, Li J, You H, Tulson G, Dang X, Song Y, Yimiti T, Wang J, Jones MK, McManus DP. Vaccination of dogs against *Echinococcus granulosus*, the cause of cystic hydatid disease in humans. The Journal of Infectious Diseases 2006;**194**:966-974. DOI: 10.1086/506622

[29] Zhang W, McManus DP. Vaccination of dogs against *Echinococcus granulosus*: A means to control hydatid disease?. Trends in Parasitology. 2008;**24**:419-424. DOI: 10.1016/j.pt.2008.05.008

[30] Torgerson PR. Dogs, vaccines and *Echinococcus*. Trends in Parasitology. 2009;**25**:57-58. DOI: 10.1016/j.pt.2008.10.003

[31] Kouguchi H, Matsumoto J, Nakao R, Yamano K, Oku Y, Yagi K. Characterization of a surface glycoprotein from *Echinococcus multilocularis* and its mucosal vaccine potential in dogs. PLoS One. 2013;**8**:e69821. DOI: 10.1371/journal.pone.0069821

[32] Kouguchi H, Irie T, Matsumoto J, Nakao R, Sugano Y, Oku Y, Yagi K. The timing of worm exclusion in dogs repeatedly infected with the cestode *Echinococcus multilocularis*. Journal of Helminthology. 2016;**90**:766-772. DOI: 10.1017/S0022149X15001169

[33] Gemmell MA, Lawson JR, Roberts MG. Population dynamics in echinococcosis and cysticercosis: Biological parameters of *Echinococcus granulosus* in dogs and sheep. Parasitology.1986;**92**:599-620. DOI: 10.1017/S0031182000053543

[34] World Health Organization. Global plan to combat neglected tropical diseases 2008-2015: Geneva, World Health Organization, 2007 (WHO/CDS/NTD/2007.3)

[35] Katsuno K, Burrows JN, Duncan K, Hooft van Huijsduijnen R, Kaneko T, Kita K, Mowbray CE, Schmatz D, Warner P, Slingsby BT. Hit and lead criteria in drug discovery for infectious diseases of the developing world. Nature Reviews Drug Discovery. 2015;**14**:751-758. DOI: 10.1038/nrd4683

[36] Matsumoto J, Sakamoto K, Shinjyo N, Kido Y, Yamamoto N, Yagi K, Miyoshi H, Nonaka N, Katakura K, Kita K, Oku Y. Anaerobic NADH-Fumarate Reductase System Is Predominant

in the Respiratory Chain of *Echinococcus multilocularis*, Providing a Novel Target for the Chemotherapy of Alveolar Echinococcosis. Antimicrob. Agents Chemotherapy. 2008;**52**: 164-170. DOI: 10.1128/AAC.00378-07

[37] Kita K, Shiomi K, Omura S. Advances in drug discovery and biochemical studies. Trends in Parasitology. 2007;**23**:223-229. DOI: 10.1016/j.pt.2007.03.005

[38] Sakai C, Tomitsuka E, Esumi H, Harada S, Kita K. Mitochondrial fumarate reductase as a target of chemotherapy: From parasites to cancer cells. Biochimica et Biophysica Acta. 2012;**1820**:643-651. DOI: 10.1016/j.bbagen.2011.12.013

[39] Inaoka DK, Shiba T, Sato D, Balogun EO, Sasaki T, Nagahama M, Oda M, Matsuoka S, Ohmori J, Honma T, Inoue M, Kita K, Harada S. Structural insights into the molecular design of flutolanil derivatives targeted for fumarate respiration of parasite mitochondria. International Journal of Molecular Sciences. 2015;**16**:15287-15308. DOI: 10.3390/ijms160715287

[40] Yamashita T, Ino T, Miyoshi H, Sakamoto K, Osanai A, Nakamaru-Ogiso E, Kita K. Rhodoquinone reaction site of mitochondrial complex I, in parasitic helminth, *Ascaris suum*. Biochimica et Biophysica Acta. 2004;**1608**:97-103. DOI: 10.1016/j.bbabio.2003.10.006

[41] Iwata F, Shinjyo N, Amino H, Sakamoto K, Islam MK, Tsuji N, Kita K. Change of subunitcomposition of mitochondrial complex II (succinate-ubiquinone reductase/quinol-fumarate reductase) in *Ascaris suum* during the migration in the experimental host. Parasitology International. 2008;**57**:54-61. DOI: 10.1016/j.parint.2007.08.002

[42] Osanai A, Harada S, Sakamoto K, Shimizu H, Inaoka DK, Kita K. Crystallization of mitochondrial rhodoquinol-fumarate reductase from the parasitic nematode *Ascaris suum* with the specific inhibitor flutolanil. Acta Crystallographica. 2009;**65**:941-944. DOI: 10.1107/S1744309109031352

[43] Miyadera H, Shiomi K, Ui H, Yamaguchi Y, Masuma R, Tomoda H, Miyoshi H, Osanai A, Kita K, Omura S. Atpenins, potent and specific inhibitors of mitochondrial complex II (succinate-ubiquinone oxidoreductase). Proceedings of the National Academy of the Sciences USA. 2003;**21**:473-477. DOI: 10.1073/pnas.0237315100

[44] Harada S, Inaoka DK, Ohmori J, and Kita K. Diversity of parasite complex II. Biochimica et Biophysica Acta. 2013;**1827**:658-667. DOI: 10.1016/j.bbabio.2013.01.005

[45] Kutik S, Rissler M, Guan XL, Guiard B, Shui G, Gebert N, Heacock PN, Rehling P, Dowhan W, Wenk MR, Pfanner N, Wiedemann N. The translocator maintenance protein Tam41 is required for mitochondrial cardiolipin biosynthesis. The Journal of Cell Biology. 2008;**183**:1213-1221. DOI: 10.1083/jcb.200806048

[46] Roos MH, Tielens AG. Differential expression of two succinate dehydrogenase subunit-B genes and a transition in energy metabolism during the development of the parasitic nematode *Haemonchus contortus*. Molecular and Biochemical Parasitology. 1994;**66**:273-281. DOI: 10.1016/0166-6851(94)90154-6

[47] Cecchini G, Schroder, I, Gunsalus RP, Maklashina E. Succinate dehydrogenase and fumarate reductase from *Escherichia coli*. Biochimica et Biophysica Acta. 2002;**1553**:140-157. DOI: 10.1016/S0005-2728(01)00238-9

[48] Ghezzi D, Goffrini P, Uziel G, Horvath R, Klopstock T, Lochmüller H, D'Adamo P, Gasparini P, Strom TM, Prokisch H, Invernizzi F, Ferrero I, Zeviani M. SDHAF1, encoding a LYR complex-II specific assembly factor, is mutated in SDH-defective infantile leukoencephalopathy. Nature Genetics. 2009;**41**:654-656. DOI: 10.1038/ng.378

[49] Hao HX, Khalimonchuk O, Schraders M, Dephoure N, Bayley JP, Kunst H, Devilee P, Cremers CW, Schiffman JD, Bentz BG, Gygi SP, Winge DR, Kremer H, Rutter J. SDH5, a gene required for flavination of succinate dehydrogenase, is mutated in paraganglioma. *Science*. 2009;**28**:1139-1142. DOI: 10.1126/science.1175689

[50] Bezawork-Geleta A, Dong L, Rohlena J, Neuzil J. The assembly factor SDHAF2 is dispensable for flavination of the catalytic subunit of mitochondrial complex II in breast cancer cells. The Journal of Biological Chemistry. 2016;**pii**: jbc.C116.755017. DOI: 10.1074/jbc.C116.755017

[51] Tsai IJ, Zarowiecki M, Holroyd N, Garciarrubio A, Sanchez-Flores A, Brooks KL, Tracey A, Bobes RJ, Fragoso G, Sciutto E, Aslett M, Beasley H, Bennett HM, Cai J, Camicia F, Clark R, Cucher M, De Silva N, Day TA, Deplazes P, Estrada K, Fernández C, Holland PW, Hou J, Hu S, Huckvale T, Hung SS, Kamenetzky L, Keane JA, Kiss F, Koziol U, Lambert O, Liu K, Luo X, Luo Y, Macchiaroli N, Nichol S, Paps J, Parkinson J, Pouchkina-Stantcheva N, Riddiford N, Rosenzvit M, Salinas G, Wasmuth JD, Zamanian M, Zheng Y, Cai X, Soberón X, Olson PD, Laclette JP, Brehm K, Berriman M. The genomes of four tapeworm species reveal adaptations to parasitism. Nature. 2013;**496**:57-63. DOI: 10.1038/nature12031

[52] Goodman CD, Siregar JE, Mollard V, Vega-Rodríguez J, Syafruddin D, Matsuoka H, Matsuzaki M, Toyama T, Sturm A, Cozijnsen A, Jacobs-Lorena M, Kita K, Marzuki S, McFadden GI. Parasites resistant to the antimalarial atovaquone fail to transmit by mosquitoes. Science. 2016;**352**:349-353. DOI: 10.1126/science.aad9279

[53] Dougherty DA. Cation-pi interactions in chemistry and biology: A new view of benzene, Phe, Tyr, and Trp. Science. 1996;**271**:163-168. DOI: 10.1126/science.271.5246.163

[54] Tóth G, Murphy RF, Lovas S. Stabilization of local structures by pi-CH and aromatic-backbone amide interactions involving prolyl and aromatic residues. Protein Engineering, Design and Selection. 2001;**14**:543-547. DOI: 10.1093/protein/14.8.543

[55] Yabu Y, Suzuki T, Nihei C, Minagawa N, Hosokawa T, Nagai K, Kita K, Ohta N. Chemotherapeutic efficacy of ascofuranone in Trypanosoma vivax-infected mice without glycerol. Parasitology International. 2006;**55**:39-43. DOI: 10.1016/j.parint.2005.09.003

[56] Kido Y, Sakamoto K, Nakamura K, Harada M, Suzuki T, Yabu Y, Saimoto H, Yamakura F, Ohmori D, Moore AL, Harada S, Kita K. Purification and kinetic characterization of recombinant alternative oxidase from *Trypanosoma brucei brucei*. Biochimica et Biophysica Acta. 2010;**1797**:443-445. DOI: 10.1016/j.bbabio.2009.12.021